ANTI-INFLAMMATORY DIET

The Complete Beginners Guide to Heal the Immune System, Feel Better, and Restore Optimal Health

(With Delicious Meal Plan to Get You Started)

&

THE ANTI-INFLAMMATORY COMPLETE COOKBOOK:

Over 100 Delicious Recipes to Reduce Inflammation, Be Healthy and Feel Amazing

ANTI-INFLAMMATORY DIET

Table of Contents

THE ANTI-INFLAMMATORY COMPLETE COOKBOOK:

Table of Contents

Introduction

Congratulations on downloading *Anti-Inflammatory Diet: The Complete Beginners Guide to Heal The Immune System, Feel Better, and Restore Optimal Health (With Delicious Meal Plan to Get You Started)* and thank you for doing so. Receiving a chronic inflammation diagnosis may seem like the end of the world but you can work through it, and picking up this book and others like it is the first step to drastically improve your quality of life going forward.

It is important to understand that when it comes to changing your diet in ways that are effective at combating inflammation, nothing is black and white. If the thought of losing your favorite food is a deal breaker, continue eating it, though moderation might be a wise choice. It is all about deciding on how much pain you want to live with and then acting on that choice. If you are interested in decreasing your pain levels a little, or a lot, then the following chapters are packed full of useful tips for helping you start and maintain a healthier diet moving forward.

This book contains proven steps and strategies designed to ensure you have the tools to moderate your symptoms as much as possible without resorting to medications or additional treatments. After discussing the specifics, there are additional chapters related to dealing with finding inflammation-friendly food in the wild as well as a 14-day complete meal plan to give you an idea of what to expect moving forward.

If, as you are working to change your diet, you slip up and backslide a little, it is important to not beat yourself up over it, and instead, consider how much healthier you are compared to when you started. The only time you should feel guilty about a dieting mistake is when you use it as an excuse to make additional unhealthy choices moving forward. Keep up the good work and remember that every day you eat healthily is a day you are actively improving your condition.

With so many choices out there when it comes to consuming this type of content, it is appreciated that you've chosen this one. Plenty of care and effort went into ensuring it contains as many interesting and useful tidbits as possible. Please enjoy!

CHAPTER 1

Understanding Inflammation

When outside forces attack your body, like a virus or bacteria, your body produces various substances and white blood cells to help protect the body against these foreign invaders. This is known as inflammation and it can be very beneficial for the healing process. However, there are certain diseases that make your body think it needs these healers but there is nothing there for them to protect against. This is when they turn on the body.

These diseases are called "autoimmune diseases" such as arthritis. Your immune system, which is normally there to protect your body, ends up damaging yourself in the response to these diseases. It does not know that the tissue is actually healthy and begins breaking it down and responding to it like it is abnormal. This is called "chronic inflammation."

There are a few challenges associated with inflammation. Mostly because inflammation is a helpful and necessary process for your body, so detecting it in your body does not mean it is chronic and not all forms of the disease are related to inflammation. For example, not all arthritis is related to chronic inflammation. The types typically associated with inflammation are gouty arthritis, psoriatic arthritis, and rheumatoid arthritis. Conditions not normally associated with inflammation include muscular pain, lower back problems, fibromyalgia, and osteoarthritis. These painful conditions affect the joints in many instances but are separate from inflammation. So how do you tell the difference?

There are clear symptoms of inflammation. For example, if you have trouble moving your joints, and they appear red and feel warm, it can be a sign of inflammation. Other times, your joints may be stiff or painful. It is common to have only one side effect or just a couple. In other cases, depending on where in your body inflammation is present, you can feel symptoms like the flu. You can contract a low fever and become chilled. Other times, you may feel exhausted or have little energy. Some patients experience a loss of appetite and headaches. It is also to have stiff muscles, not just joints. Again, these can appear as a single side effect or in combination with multiple side effects.

Causes of Inflammation

Immune system: The immune system is a common inflammation trigger as it is used to protect the body from outside influences. If the body is under attack, white blood cells are sent to the afflicted area to protect the body from whatever the threat is perceived to be. If your tissue needs protecting, white blood cells get to work secreting chemicals that cause the tissue to swell in an attempt to prevent anything else from getting into the afflicted area.

While this is fine in the short-term, if it proceeds unchecked indefinitely, as it does in those who deal with joint inflammation, it can cause aggressive swelling that can wear down the body's protections, leading to increased pain and eventually, even additional health issues if left untreated indefinitely.

If you believe you are suffering from chronic inflammation, then it is recommended that you seek out medical advice as soon as possible. There are varieties of tests that can be used in this situation including things like:

- A full physical exam

- Detailed study of existing medical history

- Checklist of common problem areas compared to existing joint stiffness

- Blood tests

- X-rays

- Observation of additional symptoms

Autoimmune disease: When disease causes inflammation of the organs, it is considered an autoimmune disease. The side effects that come along with the inflammation are going to vary based on the affected organ. If the heart is affected, then high blood pressure, shortness of breath, and the retention of fluid is common, though shortness of breath is also common if the lungs are inflamed as well. Kidney inflammation is also known to cause high blood pressure and pain is a symptom in many cases as well. Pain will not always be a symptom of inflammation, however, as many organs lack the nerve sensitivity to feel pain.

Diet: While inflammation can be caused by a wide variety of environmental concerns, one of the most common ways that most people increase their inflammation level is based on the foods they eat. It's not all bad, however, as just as there are foods that serve to fan inflammation, there are others that make it easier for the body to tell the difference between a true threat and a false alarm.

Two common perpetrators in the Standard American Diet are refined sugars and saturated fats. While fat and sugar are not necessarily harmful on their own, where they are sourced make a huge difference in the levels of inflammation they generate. For example, those living in the Mediterranean tend to eat far more omega-3 fatty acids and polyunsaturated fats and get most of their sugar from fruits and they have some of the lowest levels of inflammation, on average, of anyone in the world.

Stable glucose and blood sugar levels are also important, as high levels of both have been shown to lead to chronic inflammation. This can be seen in the fact that a majority of those who suffer from type-2 diabetes are chronically inflamed. As this only leads to additional health issues, this is why stabilizing these levels is so important to remain healthy in the long-term.

Another common cause of inflammation when it comes to diet is from food allergies whose symptoms are so mild that they go unnoticed for years if not decades. Two common food allergies that tend to go undiagnosed are to the gluten found in wheat and dairy. While this may lead to indigestion at the moment, it may also be causing serious inflammatory side effects throughout the body. Luckily, for some people, these sorts of allergies don't always mean cutting out the problem food entirely, as sometimes, it will be possible to balance things out with enough probiotics to neutralize the problem.

Generally speaking, foods that are full of additives or are especially rich are going to be the ones that are the most taxing on your body, and thus the ones causing the greatest amount of inflammation, especially when they are consumed regularly. This is due to the fact that it takes far more effort to digest a meal that is high in unhealthy elements than it does one that is full of the items discussed in the later part of this book. Over time, this causes your system to wear down more quickly than would otherwise be the case, increasing the overall amount of chronic inflammation your body experiences significantly. This leads to issues with your metabolism as well as your gut, both of which are a welcome invitation for chronic inflammation.

Physical activities: In addition to diet, improving the amount of sleep, you get each night, minimizing unhealthy physical exertions and keeping stress to a minimum are all excellent ways to ensure you keep extra inflammation to a minimum. While medications may be necessary once you develop an inflammatory disease, you can help the healing process or even prevent the development of diseases including diseases like Alzheimer's disease or cardiovascular disease by changing your diet choices.

When it comes to dealing with stress, it is especially likely to contribute to inflammation if things have progressed to the point where you feel your pulse racing, you wake up soaked with sweat, or you regularly have panic attacks. If this is the case, then the elevated levels of cortisol in your system are most likely increasing your overall inflammation level. Additional cortisol is released into your system whenever you feel threatened, either emotionally or physically, in preparation for a flight or fight response which means that if you find yourself feeling a heightened sense of anxiety or stress than normal, then your immune system is likely working overtime to keep things functioning as close to normal as possible, creating even more chronic inflammation in the process.

Physical stress causes much the same effects, though only certain types will trigger additional inflammation. The physical stress you are looking to avoid is the type that is caused when your body senses that it is in physical danger. While this doesn't sound difficult at first, it becomes much trickier for some people when they realize that the body takes a lack of vital nutrients as a life-threatening situation. This means that if you want to reduce your physical stress, improving your diet is a great place to start.

If your nutritional needs are not met for a prolonged period of time, it is possible that you could develop an imbalance in your GI tract which can lead to a host of additional issues. It can also cause other physical issues including hives. If these needs aren't met for a truly prolonged period of time, it can even cause your body to start shutting down completely. While it may not seem like it at the time, this is actually the body's way of protecting itself, as it is the only way that it can ensure vital organs continue to get the nutrients and energy they need to keep functioning.

While everyone has a certain level of chronic inflammation in their body at all times, you will likely not experience any negative side effects as long as it is in the low tier of severity. However, over time, you will likely begin to notice the side effects of untreated inflammation. This is why it is so important to remain vigilant and do everything in your power to ensure you remain as inflammation free as possible.

Gastrointestinal tract: It is only natural for inflammation to start in the gut as this is where nutrients are absorbed from the foods you eat. Luckily, the gut is one of the most sensitive parts of the body when it comes to inflammation which means that if your gut is inflamed, it is unlikely that you won't know about it. Common symptoms that your gut is inflamed include pain, diarrhea, constipation, flatulence, and bloating. Addressing what you eat, say by following an anti-inflammation diet, is a great way to improve the health of your gut and decrease inflammation throughout the body as well.

Due to this higher than average level of sensitivity, these types of issues tend to serve as an early warning sign against inflammation if you learn how to listen to them. In fact, with practice, you may find that the turmoil you experience is enough to properly diagnose, and thus treat, the problems you are experiencing. The anti-inflammatory diet is particularly useful in this regard as it encourages an increase in fat consumption and probiotic intake, two things proven to readily deal with these types of issues. Along with this change, extra exercise is a great way to jumpstart your GI tract and gets things working normally once more.

Hormonal imbalance: If your body's hormones are out of whack for one reason or another, inflammation is a common result. The issues most likely to generate additional inflammation include imbalances to certain levels of progesterone, testosterone, and estrogen. This is an especially common issue for women who are going through menopause, as they tend to regularly deal with a variety of hormonal imbalances.

Specific materials: Much like food allergies, some people are allergic to specific materials, typically those that are manmade such as nylon, latex, or plastic. If you have a mild allergy to one of these materials that you deal with on a regular basis, you may not even realize it is the case as the manifestation of the issue only appears as internal inflammation. If you experience periods of lightheadedness or shortness of breath that you have trouble explaining, then this could be the reason why. Similar issues can also occur if you are regularly exposed to a chemical that you are allergic to like cleaning products or scented candles. The worst offenders in this category are things that can be absorbed through the skin either intentionally or unintentionally. These chemicals can exist in the water and air, at your work, or in your home. It is important to recognize the inflammatory symptoms so that you know what to avoid in the future.

Results of Chronic Inflammation

Chronic inflammation can cause a number of issues that might not otherwise be obvious at first glance; this is what makes it so insidious, however, as it is difficult to fight something that is so hard to see. Being aware of the following facts about inflammation may make it easier to see the effects it is having on you every day, which in turn, will make them easier to rally against and eradicate once and for all.

Gut damage: Many of the immune cells that the body uses to fight off inflammation naturally group in clusters around and in the intestines where they largely ignore the bacteria living and working there. Occasionally, however, this truce breaks down and the immune cells attack the bacteria, causing a form of chronic inflammation that is responsible for many common gastrointestinal issues. If this inflammation is left untreated, the immune cells will eventually start attacking the digestive tract which can lead to irritable bowel disease, ulcerative colitis, or even Crohn's disease. Additional symptoms may include ulcers, cramps, and diarrhea and may require intestinal removal to treat properly.

Joint damage: If inflammation occurs in the joints for a prolonged period of time, it can lead to numerous serious and painful issues, the first and foremost of which is rheumatoid arthritis. This autoimmune disease occurs when, much like in the gut scenario above, the body starts attacking the otherwise health joints after enough untreated inflammation has occurred in the area to render it unrecognizable to its own defenders. If left untreated for long enough, rheumatoid arthritis can spread throughout the body and even cause vision issues later in life.

Cardiovascular damage: The type of diet that is likely to promote inflammation is also likely to create fatty buildup in the arteries which can lead to chronic inflammation as well as damaged blood cells. This inflammation is then known to attract immune cells and other white blood cells in an effort to repair the damaged area.

Unable to do so, the collection of cells can then become a clot which can directly lead to a heart attack or other cardiovascular issues. Unfortunately, even those who do not otherwise seem at risk for heart problems can experience these issues unexpectedly if their diet is full of stealthy inflammatory foods.

Cancer risk: When inflammation of a chronic variety occurs in certain vulnerable locations including the digestive tract, cervix, esophagus, or lungs, then that inflammation can lead to the formation of cancer cells. In fact, those with high levels of inflammation have been known to have nearly a 70 percent greater chance of getting cancer in their lifetime. Any time chronic inflammation is allowed to continue unchecked, immune regulation is going to break down and that is the environment that cancer is known to proliferate most rapidly in.

Hurts your sleep: Studies show that the higher the level of inflammation that a subject experienced, the less likely that they were to get the proper amount of sleep each night which is estimated to be roughly 7.6 hours each night. It is unclear if the increased levels of inflammation cause sleep-related issues or if it is the other way around. The one thing that is clear is those that are chronically unable to get enough sleep are likely to experience higher than average levels of stress and lower than average general immune systems which ultimately opens them up to a wider variety of diseases than their healthier counterparts.

Lung damage: When chronic inflammation is allowed to continue unchecked in the lungs, it can cause several types of issues including an increase in overall fluid accumulation or a general narrowing of the airway, both of which can make it much more difficult than normal to draw breath properly. This, in turn, can lead to chronic obstructive pulmonary disease as well as asthma, chronic bronchitis, and emphysema. Inflammation in the lungs is brought about by the usual causes as well as eating an excessive amount of cured meat, long periods of obesity, many common household cleaners, air pollution, and smoking cigarettes.

Gum damage: When chronic inflammation is allowed to progress for a prolonged period in the mouth, it typically starts by damaging the gums through the disease known as periodontitis which is caused by a large accumulation of bacteria there. This then causes the gums to erode, which then exposes the support structure of the teeth themselves which is will be damaged and permanently weakened. Omega-3 fatty acids are a great way to prevent chronic inflammation in general, but periodontitis specifically. If left untreated for long enough, periodontal issues can spread beyond mere oral health and can lead to an increased risk of heart disease and even dementia.

Causes weight loss issues: Those who are already obese are likely to see a higher rate of inflammation throughout the body. This increased inflammation rate can actually make it more difficult to take the weight off and keep it off because many of the proteins that are present in those with high inflammation levels are actual weight loss inhibitors. As a result, chronic inflammation is known to decrease the metabolism, which at the same time, increasing the number of hunger signals that the brain receives. At the same time, it is also known to decrease insulin resistance which makes those who are overweight and chronically inflamed more likely to develop diabetes and also gain the weight back again in the future, even if they managed to initially take it off.

Bone damage: When left untreated, chronic inflammation is known to make it more difficult for natural bone growth to occur. While this seems as though it would only affect the young, in reality, parts of the skeletal structure are naturally replaced throughout the average lifespan as they wear out through a process known as remodeling. This means that chronic inflammation can cause a decrease in bone mass, especially when left untreated for years at a time. Additionally, gastrointestinal inflammation can also lead to a decrease in bone health as it can make it difficult for the body to absorb all of the nutrients that promote proper bone health including calcium and vitamin D.

Chronic Inflammation FAQ

What increases your risk of chronic inflammation?

While all of the reasons a person may contract chronic inflammation are as of yet unclear, it is known that prolonged exposure to harsh chemicals, pesticides, or pollution can increase the risk of developing chronic inflammation. As can smoking cigarettes, being a woman, and being between the ages of 40 and 60.

What less common symptoms might appear?

While it is less common, roughly 40 percent of those with some degree of inflammation are known to experience some form of chest pain. This can include cardiovascular issues which are why it is important to monitor all chest pains carefully. Hearing loss also occurs in roughly 15 percent of those whose chronic inflammation is left untreated, while roughly 30 percent experience moderate to severe mood changes at one time or another. Depression may also occur through the specific reasons for this are widely debated.

Other potential issues include digestive issues or stomach pain which can include either diarrhea or constipation. Finally, an increased risk of broken bones and a general numbness in affected areas also occurs for some people.

What can I expect going forward?

Chronic inflammation treatments tend to vary based on how severe the inflammation is to start, its severity, previous treatment decisions, and other preferences or mitigating issues including things like daily schedule or side effects. Treatment options will then be presented in an effort to prevent serious disability, decrease the rate of permanent damage, and mitigate pain while ensuring the lifestyle of the person with inflammation changes as little as possible.

Once a plan has been formed, it will include a multi-step approach including a number of initial medicines to mitigate the most pressing issues. This will be followed up with a discussion of lifelong care options including dietary and exercise concerns as well as regular checkups which will monitor things like the number of inflamed joints, increase in muscle stiffness, and overall levels of pain. Surgery may be an option when primary joints including the feet, knees, and hips may be severely affected. Surgery options can include everything up to complete joint replacement.

What are the common treatments?

Seeking the care of a physician and discussing a mix of medication and lifestyle changes is always the best option. Many people find substantial relief from natural solutions related to diet and more. Besides a healthier diet, those with chronic inflammation tend to find some relief from their inflammation symptoms simply by taking more frequent breaks during the day so as to give their tired body's some relief.

That is not to say that exercise has no place in the life of those with chronic inflammation. Exercising the right way is considered a core part of the common chronic inflammation treatment plan and it frequently emphasizes things like flexibility and muscle strengthening programs as well as low-impact aerobics and even yoga. Exercise sessions are often capped with warm baths or heating pads to sooth problem areas or cold treatments to mitigate instances of precise pain.

Topical treatments come in a variety of forms, all of which are applied to the afflicted areas directly. These are often used in conjunction with things like physical therapies and natural treatments. Relaxation and breathing techniques have been shown to do wonders for some types of deep pain and some types of stretching and even acupuncture has been shown to help with joint stiffness. Acupressure has also been shown to have many of the same effects for those who are not fond of needles.

What can cause inflammation to worsen?

Chronic inflammation is known to increase in severity if the person in question has a cyclic citrullinated peptide in their system. Another strong indicator is if early pain proves to initially be resistant to therapy. An influx of additional joint symptoms or an extreme loss of cartilage or bone mass also indicates an especially severe case.

Inflammation is known to cause an increased collection of plaque to form on the arteries. Additional conditions which worsen this state seem to have an adverse effect when it comes to inflammation as well. If not treated, this can lead to an increase in the risk of a heart attack as well as a stroke.

Is surgery an effective option?

The effectiveness in treating chronic inflammation with surgery depends on the severity of the condition as well as the joints affected. Larger joints can be completely replaced in an effort to restore a majority of previous levels of movement, though this surgery often requires a good deal of physical therapy afterward. A variety of surgeries can be done to remove inflamed tissue, but this only treats the issue, it will not cure it. In addition, these types of surgeries can be difficult to perform on smaller joints.

Is pain while exercising normal?

Exercise is an important part of dealing with chronic inflammation, but that doesn't mean it will be a painless process. Especially when first getting started, it is common for those with inflammation to experience pain and soreness. Despite this, it is likely to produce long-term relief from pain and is strongly encouraged. If you find that you are still experiencing pain after the six-week mark, consider modifying the amount and type of exercise you are participating in. Ensure you always use proper cool down and warmup techniques and that you are wearing appropriate shoes for the occasion.

When some pain is normal, a significant increase in swelling or a red hot burning feeling is the signs that you should see a doctor. It is also important to be aware of the pain that does not go away with time or other treatments or that lingers for more than two hours after the exercise has finished. Finally, pain that results in limping or is otherwise constant sharp or stabbing should also be considered a warning sign.

How exactly does body weight affect chronic inflammation?

While many of the factors surrounding chronic inflammation are still rather vague, studies show that striving to maintain a healthy weight for your height directly correlates to a lower chance of contracting inflammation, and for those with the disease, a direct correlation to a decrease of additional flare-ups. A loss of just five percent of a person's body weight is enough to significantly reduce chronic pain as well as potential debilitation.

How is inflammation different than Osteoarthritis?

Osteoarthritis is caused by long-term stress and general wear placed on the joints as people age. As such, it occurs more slowly and appears in older people than the range that chronic inflammation targets. In terms of presentation of symptoms, osteoarthritis typically causes joints to ache but there is rarely any swelling. Stiffness may also occur though it typically lasts less than an hour in the morning; it may also reappear in the evenings.

How does inflammation differ from Psoriatic Arthritis?

Chronic inflammation and psoriatic arthritis are quite similar as both are caused by immune system malfunction and result in inflammation. Unlike chronic inflammation, psoriatic arthritis presents symptoms of psoriatic lesions on the skin and rarely affects joints symmetrically. In addition, chronic inflammation frequently presents more swelling than psoriatic arthritis does. Psoriatic arthritis is more common in adults who are already suffering from psoriasis.

CHAPTER 2

Anti-Inflammatory Diet Breakdown

While there is no magic bullet when it comes to lowering your inflammation, it is important to eat a healthy and balanced diet that is at least 60 percent of vegetables, fruits, and whole grains. The remainder should come from lean protein and low-fat dairy. To be as proactive as possible, it is important to consider what you are regularly putting into your body as well as specific foods to avoid.

The anti-inflammatory diet is not a diet in the modern sense of the word as its primary focus is not to help people lose weight, though it is a healthy way of eating so it is certainly possible to lose weight while sticking to the guidelines outlined below. Instead, it is more of a lifestyle choice based on the scientific data available regarding the foods that are known to increase inflammation and those that are known to decrease it. In addition to helping you decrease the build-up of inflammation in your body, the anti-inflammatory diet will also help you look and feel better than you have in years thanks to the energy and ancillary health benefits that come along with a diet high in phytonutrients, dietary fiber, essential fatty acids, minerals, and vitamins.

Foods That Help Fight Inflammation

Omega-3 fatty acids commonly found in fish oil is a natural anti-inflammatory nutrient that is known to occur in higher amounts in tuna, salmon, trout, mackerel, and herring when compared to other cold-water fish. Fish oil has been shown to ease morning stiffness as well as relive some of the pain caused by tender joints. There is roughly 1 gram of Omega-3 per 3.5 oz. of fish and supplements are also available. It is important to talk to your doctor for a target amount of Omega-3 per day as ingesting too much has been known to interfere with certain types of medications.

Fiber: Vegetables, fruits, and whole grains all contain fiber which has been shown to reduce inflammation. The amount of fiber that those dealing with inflammation consume can be directly correlated to a lower level of C-reactive protein, a strong indicator of inflammation levels.

Oil: Both of the coconut and olive oil varieties are known to decrease inflammation in a similar fashion to both aspirin and ibuprofen. Both are high in oleocanthal which interacts with the enzymes responsible for creating inflammation and slows their process.

Supplements: Those who are suffering from inflammation typically have low levels of selenium, which can be found in abundance in whole grains as well as crab, oysters, and other shellfish. Unfortunately, high amounts of selenium are known to be linked to diabetes so it is important to discuss these types of supplements with your doctor. Vitamin D has also been shown to help lower the inflammation risk in women as it helps improve the immune system in general. Vitamin D can be found in low-fat milk, whole grains, and eggs.

Foods to Avoid

Omega-6 fatty acids are typically found in soybeans, corn, and sunflower seeds as well as fried foods and most snack foods. Omega-6 is the opposite of omega-3 in that it increases the risk of obesity as well as inflammation.

Vitamins and minerals: that are required for a healthy immune system are often depleted during inflammation treatment. As such, those with inflammation need to be sure to monitor their zinc, magnesium, calcium, vitamin E, vitamin B12, vitamin B6, vitamin D, vitamin C, and folic acid. A good choice is to up your vegetable intake as a result as it is important to not rely too heavily on supplements.

Anti-Inflammation Guidelines

- Ensure you consume a minimum of 5 vegetables per day; ensure they encompass the color spectrum whenever possible.

- Ensure you consume at least 5 servings of healthy fats per day. This includes seeds and nuts as well as coconut or olive oil.

- Ensure you consume at least 4 fruits per day and stick with fibrous fruits for at least 3 of those.

- Ensure you consume at least 3 servings or cracked or whole grains per day, the more full of seeds the better.

- Ensure you consume at least 1 serving of beans per day, there are plenty of different types of beans out there, try a variety.

- Ensure you consume no more than 2 servings of al dente pasta per week.

- Ensure you consume at least 4 servings of fish per week.

- Ensure you consume beef no more than 2 times per week.

- You are free to drink up to 4 glasses of oolong, green or white tea per day.

- Up to two glass of red wine per day has been shown to help inflammation.

Diet Tips

Don't discount variety: When following an anti-inflammatory diet, there is no reason you should fail to experience as much variety in your day to day diet like anyone else. However, as with any new diet, early on, it can be easy for you to find a handful of things that you like and stick with them, simply because finding new things to eat may seem intimidating.

This is not recommended; however, as following the anti-inflammatory diet is more about building a new and improved healthy lifestyle, something that won't be possible if you never try anything new. As such, a good way of broadening your horizon is to eat something that is green, something that is red, and something that is orange at every meal. Foods that are these colors tend to naturally be healthier and full of more filling nutritional content than the alternative. What's more, these foods are often credited with making those who eat them look and feel younger as well.

Drink more water: Since you are adding new habits to your repertoire anyway, it is a good idea to add drinking more water to the list. Specifically, you should aim for about 64 ounces of water per day, to ensure your body has all the water it needs to operate at maximum efficiency. If you live in a warm, dry climate, or exercise regularly, you are going to want to aim even higher and try and consume a gallon of water per day. If you don't drink that much water naturally or don't believe you need to drink the recommended amount, give it a try for a few weeks and you will be surprised by the results.

Specifically, you will be surprised at how frequently your body was sending you signals saying it was hungry when in reality it was just looking for something to drink. Drinking the right amount of water per day will also provide your metabolism with the boost that it needs to function in peak form and ensure you lose as much weight each week as possible.

Avoid processed foods: While it should come as no surprise that following the anti-inflammatory diet means cutting out certain foods, the reality is often more difficult for many people than they first anticipated. The fact of the matter is, giving up processed foods with their high amount of unhealthy fats and sugars, can be just as difficult as quitting smoking as your body has long become accustomed to the steady flow of these pleasure-inducing substances. This means you will likely experience a decrease in your general energy levels and may even experience symptoms commonly associated with the flu. This is nothing to worry about, however, and it is just your body adjusting to your new and improved lifestyle. Stick with it and you will soon feel healthier than you have in years.

Processed foods are any that are either chemically treated or are made of ingredients that have been refined or are artificially created. The food you are looking for should instead be as free of chemicals as possible and only made from pure, unrefined ingredients. When it comes to comparing the two types of food, as a rule, the processed versions are practically guaranteed to have roughly twice as much sugar as their natural counterparts. Sugar consumption should be limited when consumed as part of a healthy diet for the way that it can negatively influence the metabolism.

The amount of sugar added to processed foods only serve to make them seem more appealing to the unaware consumer thanks to an ancient affinity to sugar built-in from the days when humanity was nothing more than hunter-gatherers. In those times, items that were high in fat and sugar content were typically high in healthy vitamins and nutrients as well. Modern companies are aware of this connection and, as such, pump their products full of these things to get consumers to eat more than ever.

What's worse, the high amount of sugar and unhealthy fats in modern processed foods are of high enough levels that the human body can become physically addicted to them, which is why it is possible to eat an entire bag of fast food and still be craving more.

The human body is programmed to never get enough fat and sugar. Consuming too much can leave the brain unable to produce the types of pleasure generating chemicals the food supplies naturally and can lead to serious withdrawal symptoms if cut out cold turkey.

As a good rule of thumb, remember, foods that are high in preservatives, flavorings, additives, coloring, or texture additives should be ignored at all costs. Refined carbohydrates are also a strong warning sign and will only produce a fraction of the energy that their complex cousins can in the same servings.

Know your ideal calorie intake: When your body is at rest, the rate at which your body is using energy is the Basal Metabolic Rate or BMR for short. To carry out the simplest of bodily functions such as breathing and digesting food, your body will burn a certain number of calories every day. This obviously means your body needs to intake at least that specific number of calories unless you want it to quit functioning properly. Here are a couple of ways to determine your body's specific caloric need:

To determine your basal metabolic rate, use this equation:

For an average woman

(4.7 x your height in inches) + (4.35 x your weight in pounds) - (4.7 x your age in years) + 65

For an average man

(12.7 x your height in inches) + (6.23 x your weight in pounds) - (6.8 x your age in years) + 66

The math will help you to determine the calories your body needs just to continue breathing. If you do more than just lie in bed all day, your body will need a bit more calories than provided. The above formulas can now be multiplied by your activity level. The answer to these equations will give you a rough idea of your daily caloric need.

- If you exercise very rarely, multiply your BMR by 1.2.

- If you exercise lightly 1-3 times a week, multiply your BMR by 1.375.

- If you exercise moderately 3-5 times a week, multiply your BMR by 1.55.

- If you play sports or exercise hard 6-7 times a week, multiply your BMR by 1.725.

- If you work a very physically demanding job or work out twice a week or more, multiply your BMR by 1.9.

For example, a woman desiring to determine her essential caloric requirements using this method would do the following:

$(4.7 \times 64.5) + (4.35 \times 137) - (4.7 \times 29) + 65 = 1417.8$

The solution here is her basal metabolic rate. This tells her that she needs to eat 1417.8 calories a day simply to survive.

In addition to knowing the number of calories you should consume per day, it is important to know the combination of macronutrients

Know your macros: In addition to knowing how many calories you should aim to consume per day, it is also important to ensure you are consuming the right combination of macronutrients, carbs, fats, and proteins each day as well.

- **Ectomorph:** If you're an ectomorph, you're naturally thin with skinny limbs with a high tolerance for carbohydrates. Usually, your metabolic rate is fast. Ectomorphs are typically built so they have long limbs and smaller muscles in their core. Even if they do put on weight, they will still tend to look skinnier than they are in both their forearms and calves. This doesn't mean that they are always weak, however, and they can certainly put on muscle like anyone else, they just need to consume far more healthy calories in order to do so successfully. A good starting macronutrient ratio for you would be something like 25 percent protein, 55 percent carbs, and 20 percent fat.

- **Mesomorph:** Mesomorphs are naturally muscular and athletic. They have a moderate carbohydrate tolerance and a moderate metabolic rate. They have moderate metabolisms and their bodies prefer to build muscle and maintain a lower overall level of fat. Mesomorphs can usually start at a 30 percent protein, 40 percent carb, and 30 percent fat macronutrient ratio.

- **Endomorph:** If you're naturally broad and thick, you're probably an endomorph. They tend to be larger than the other body types, simply because their metabolism is slower, so they more readily hang onto fat as well as muscle. Endomorphs have a low carbohydrate tolerance and a slow metabolic rate. If you're an endomorph, try a ratio of 35 percent protein, 25 percent carbs, and 40 percent fat.

CHAPTER 3

Making the Transition

Getting Started

If you find yourself suddenly dealing with chronic inflammation, there will be a number of choices you are going to have to make when it comes to dietary changes. It is important to understand that this does not mean you have to give up your favorite foods; you will just have to accept the additional discomfort that comes along with consuming them. The first thing you will need to determine if you are sensitive to gluten and if this sensitivity affects your inflammation. A gluten sensitivity rules out barley, rye, and wheat, in addition to all other products commonly made from traditional flour or refined grains.

You will need to learn to look at labels and determine which processed and packaged foods you can easily consume as the list will be few and far between. Most processed or prepackaged foods contain items from the list above so it is important to memorize this list as you will be referring to it frequently. A big reason for this is because of the high amount of trans fats that comes along with being a processed food. Trans fats contain high levels of C-reactive protein and should be cut out of your diet whenever possible.

In addition, it is important to cut down on your soda intake immediately or switch to tea to wean yourself from caffeine. Even sugar-free sodas can increase inflammation so quit now, you will be glad you did. Cutting out additional unnecessary sugars is also a great idea. Replacing unhealthy snacks with healthy, inflammation-fighting snacks will also at a bit of pep to your step.

What it comes down to is that you should make it a point to increase your vegetable and fruit intake substantially, as well as things like fish, nuts, and other lean protein. Eat when you are hungry, stop when you feel full, and make sure you are consuming enough calories to remain healthy while exercising. Stick to these rules and you will find the anti-inflammation diet to be the easiest diet you have ever tried.

Chapter 6 offers up a 14-day example diet plan to show you just how varied and delicious the diet can be. If you run across something you don't like, feel free to alter it based on the options discussed above. The only thing you need to keep in mind is how you feel and how best to make sure tomorrow you feel even better.

Eating on the Go

While packing some seeds, nuts, or fruit for a midday snack on the go means you won't have to worry about finding a snack on the road, eating out with an eye towards keeping your inflammation in check, is easier than you might think. When picking a restaurant whether out and about locally, in the airport, or abroad, make selections with an eye towards ethnic flare. A wide variety of options including traditional Italian, Greek, Hispanic, Asian, and Indian food typically place a larger focus on vegetables, lean protein, and plenty of anti- inflammatory spices such as willow bark, garlic, cinnamon, turmeric, coriander, ginger, and even simple black pepper.

When compared with meals consumed at home, eating out typically includes significantly more options when it comes to processed grains which is why it is important to have an understanding of how grains, and especially gluten and lectin, affect you. The human body is not designed to handle nearly as many processed grains as the modern diet suggests. In fact, the human body hasn't really caught up to the concept of agriculture at all. As such, many people have an issue with the gluten that is found in all forms of grains and for those with inflammation, this allergy can cause inflammation flare-ups. Lectin is a mild toxin found in many grains that may also agitate inflammation symptoms.

Exercise

The level of exercise you can safely perform while dealing with your chronic inflammation will vary greatly depending on your current prognosis, symptoms you are showing, and your general level of physical fitness. Exercise is known to be especially helpful in the early stages of the condition and can help to fight off the initial feelings of fatigue that many people experience.

Exercise is useful for those who are looking to lose weight as a way to help mitigate numerous conditions that can lead to chronic inflammation in the first place. Exercise can also strengthen the heart making it less likely that cardiovascular issues will occur. It is also known to decrease instances of anxiety as well as depression.

Those who start exercising are encouraged to remember that this does not give them a free pass to eating less healthy foods as the reasons certain foods are off- limits has nothing to do with calorie counts. Ignoring dietary restrictions will only force your body to work even harder and possibly even increase the severity of existing inflammation.

What follows are a few exercises of the sort you should aim for when starting to exercise while on the anti-inflammatory diet.

- *Butterflies:* For this workout, you can stand. Bring your hands by your ears so that the elbows are bent, and bend over so that your back is flat. Next, lift the elbows away from the ears, making sure that the shoulder blades are pushing towards one another. Repeat this exercise for at least thirty reps, because of the fact that you will not be using weights. If you want to experience more intensity, using weights for this exercise will certainly intensify the workout.

- *Squats:* To do a proper squat, begin in a standing position with your arms hanging freely at your sides and your feet planted so they are even with your shoulders. Start the exercises by bending your knees while simultaneously moving your hips as if you were planning to sit in a chair and bend as far as possible. Without stopping, return to the standing position. This is a great exercise if you are interested in strengthening your core and your legs.

- *Leg drop:* To begin this exercise, you will want to lie on your back with your legs pointed up toward the ceiling. From this position, lower first one leg so that it is parallel with the ground before returning it to the starting position. Repeat with the other leg. While practicing this exercise, it is important that you always keep your leg straight. This exercise will strengthen your core.

- *Kick-ups:* To begin this exercise, you will want to get on your hands and knees so that your weight is supported by both your knees and your forearms. You will then alternate between legs as you lift one leg off of the ground and kick backward so your heels face upwards. You will then return the leg to the starting position in one fluid motion.

- *Hip Bridge:* To begin this exercise, you will want to lie on your back so that your knees are bent and both of your feet are planted firmly on the floor. You will then want to lift your hips as far off the ground as possible, while at the same time clenching your buttocks, with the end goal being to create a perfectly straight line between your knees as your shoulders.

- *Plank:* To begin this exercise, you will want to get on your hands and knees before placing all of your weight on your forearms and balancing on your toes. After you are in the position, you will then want to tense your entire body, placing special focus on your core, and hold that position for as long as possible.

- *Superman:* To perform this exercise, you will want to lay face down on the ground with your arms out in front of you and your legs straight. You will then simply lift both your arms and legs off the ground at the same time, as high as you can. During this exercise, you will want to keep your arms and legs stable rather than moving up and down, you will also want to hold for as long as possible.

- *Push-ups:* To begin this exercise, you will want to place your hands on the ground at slightly more than shoulder width and place your weight on your and toes. When you are ready, flex your core and, using only your arms, and lower yourself as close to the ground as you can manage while still being able to return to the starting position. For the best results, you are going to want to breathe in while you are going towards the ground and breathe in as you start back in the opposite direction. Additionally, rather than aiming to hit a specific number of push-ups at a time, simply keep going for as long as you can maintain proper form.

Cooking Tips

Combating sodium: When it comes to salt, practically everyone uses way more than is necessary to get the most out of the condiment. In fact, taste tests show that as little as one-eighth of a teaspoon is enough for most people to notice. Cutting out salt completely at first will cause you to feel as though everything is suddenly bland, cutting back to a firm measured amount will already go a long way toward making a positive difference.

Additionally, it is important to move away from canned items like tomatoes, broths, even beans. The juices many items are canned in are typically brimming with salt. Use fresh alternatives or make your own extremely healthy bone broth instead. In addition, it is important to always read every label as extra salt can be hiding practically anywhere. For example, the average piece of white bread has as much as 170 mg of sodium.

Instead of using additional salt as a seasoning, consider using a splash of vinegar or lemon juice to bring out the meat's natural flavors. On the other hand, instead of using a salty flavor to balance out the sourness, consider adding a pinch of something sweet instead. Likewise, instead of using salt to balance out a bitter flavor, a dash of something sweet can balance it and add extra complexity to the dish. If you are striving to make something more savory, don't reach for the salt, and instead try something which contains the amino acid known as L-glutamate, things like carrots, nuts, or mushrooms are all good choices.

While salt is an easy way to add a bit of flavor to a meal, it is not the only way to do so. Consider sautéed, toasted, and roasted alternatives to your traditional cooking methods to add a bit of extra style and taste to the meal. If you have never roasted something before, you will be surprised at how it can add an entirely new dimension to a favored dish.

Experiment with fresh herbs instead of simple salt. Dried herbs and spices have long since become the norm. Defy convention and grind your own fresh varieties instead. You will be surprised at the difference it makes. Consider using more oils and other flavorful fats in your cooking as well. In many cases, salt is simply an easy solution to a complicated problem. It will usually do well enough but it is rarely the best option. Take a few more minutes during your cooking and expand your horizons, you will never want to go back to simply salt again.

Try Superfoods: To understand just why these foods are so terrific, it is important to understand what free radicals are and how oxidation works. Oxidation is the name for the way the body uses chemical reactions to create energy. This process sometimes creates a byproduct known as a free radical.

These radicals are a form of the molecule that is unstable and can damage cell membranes, proteins, and even genes. They are known to contribute to many problematic issues including Alzheimer's disease, heart disease, cancer, the signs of aging, and many chronic diseases including chronic inflammation. The kidneys typically work to remove many of these free radicals, but if they are working in a limited capacity, these superfoods can pick up the slack. Luckily, there are plenty of superfoods to choose from.

- *Red Bell Peppers:* Red bell peppers are ideal for those suffering from chronic inflammation as they are full of fiber, folic acid, vitamin B6, vitamin C, and vitamin A while also being low in potassium. Another boon is the high concentration of lycopene, an antioxidant that will help fight inflammation across the board. Red bell peppers are great in chicken or tuna salad or simply eaten with the right dip. Roasted, they make a great addition to any salad or sandwich. They also add a mild kick to kabobs, egg dishes, or as a part of a ground turkey or beef meal.

- *Cabbage:* Cabbage is a great choice if you are looking to reduce the number of free radicals floating around and possibly damaging your system as it contains high amounts of phytochemicals which break them apart on contact. They are also known to improve cardiovascular health and fight cancer. What's more, it is a good source of folic acid, B6, fiber, vitamin C, and vitamin K. Cabbage is a great addition to fish tacos or coleslaw and can be microwaved, steamed, or boiled depending on personal preferences. It can also be eaten by itself with just a bit of cream cheese or butter.

- *Cauliflower:* Cauliflower contains numerous compounds that help the liver remove inflammation-causing toxins from the body, a boon during times when you have eaten more inflammation causing foods than you should have. It also contains lots of fiber, folate, and vitamin C. Cauliflower is delicious with a simple dip, in salads, boiled, or steamed. Cauliflower makes a great substitute for things like rice and potatoes and can be flavored in a myriad of ways.

- *Garlic:* Garlic makes a good flavor substitute for those who are watching their salt intake. It also naturally lowers cholesterol and mitigates inflammation. Garlic has fewer anti-inflammatory and anti-clotting effects once it has been cooked so it is best consumed raw for maximum results. Garlic is an appropriate salt substitute in everything from sauces to vegetables, to any type of protein.

- *Onion:* Powered onion also makes a great salt substitute in a wide variety of circumstances. In addition, it contains high amounts of a flavonoid known as quercetin which prevents fatty deposits from building up inside the body. Quercetin is also known to be a strong antioxidant that can reduce the risk of cancer and heart disease. Onions are also low in potassium and high in chromium which is beneficial whit it comes to helping the metabolism maintain proper function especially if it has been negatively affected by inflammation. They can be consumed cooked or raw with no difference in their effectiveness.

- *Apples:* Apples contain lots of fiber as well as vitamins which help to mitigate inflammation. They are also known to reduce cancer risk, prevent heart disease, help with constipation, and lower cholesterol. They are just as healthy cooked as they are raw and can also be consumed in cider or juice form.

- *Cranberries:* Cranberries are very acidic and help prevent harmful bacteria from forming in the bladder which is great for ensuring the urinary tract remains uninfected, especially if it is an area in which you regularly deal with chronic inflammation. They are also high in vitamins which can reduce heart disease or cancer risks. Cranberries are just as healthy when dried as they are when fresh and either can be added to most salads or cereals with ease.

- *Blueberries:* Blueberries are blue because they contain lots of anthocyanins, a type of compound bursting with antioxidants. This means they contain lots of fiber and vitamin C while also helping to mitigate inflammation. The manganese they contain is also great for preventing bone-related issues that may appear as a result of a calcium deficiency. Blueberries are great by themselves, dried, baked into a pastry, or with cereal.

- *Raspberries:* Raspberries are known to contain what is known as ellagic acid, a compound which is known to help destroy free radicals in the bloodstream. Their red color comes from anthocyanins, a cousin of anthocyanins which is also a strong antioxidant. They are also known to help reduce cancer cells or tumor growth.

- *Strawberries:* Strawberries contain lots of fiber, manganese, and vitamin C as well as other vitamins and minerals known to help prevent cancer, maintain heart health, and mitigate inflammation. They make a great natural desert or addition to cereal or smoothies.

- *Cherries:* Eating cherries daily has been shown to measurably reduce the amount of inflammation in chronic situations on a regular basis. They are also full of antioxidants as well as phytochemicals which help reduce the risk of heart disease. Cherries are great on their own, in desserts, and also as a sauce for either pork or lamb.

- *Red Grapes:* Red grapes get their color from the flavonoids they contain which help maintain heart health as well as reducing the risk of blood clots and improving oxidation when it comes to overall blood flow. One particular flavonoid known as resveratrol is also known to improve the amount of nitric oxide the body produces to increase relaxation of blood vessels. It is also known to reduce the risk of cancer and stop inflammation in its tracks. Choose grapes that appear more vibrant for the best results. Those who are monitoring their water intake can freeze grapes prior to eating.

- *Egg Whites:* Egg whites are literally pure protein while also containing a wealth of vital amino acids. It is also an easy way to monitor your protein intake if required. Egg whites can be eaten on their own, in salads, with tuna, and even in smoothies.

- *Mushrooms:* Mushrooms contain more vitamin D than any other vegetable or fruit which makes it a good choice for those looking to fight chronic inflammation. Mushrooms can find a natural home in salads, soups, and as a sauce for a variety of dishes.

- *Kale:* Kale is a terrific choice for those facing chronic inflammation as it is loaded with flavonoids and carotenoids both of which can reduce the risk of heart disease and cancer. It is also full of calcium, vitamin C, vitamin A, and vitamin K. Kale is a great snack choice as it can be baked and consumed as a chip.

- *Spinach:* Spinach contains a high amount of what is known as beta- carotene, an important component to consider when working in keeping your immune system as healthy as possible. It also contains lots of folates, vitamin K, vitamin C, and vitamin A. This is an ideal replacement for lettuce in most salads.

Consider the Mediterranean Diet

If you are interested in changing your diet so as to decrease your risk of inflammation but are looking for something with a few more guidelines than those listed above, consider the Mediterranean Diet. The Mediterranean Diet was created in the 1960s when it was discovered that those in the region surrounding the Mediterranean

Sea naturally live longer, healthier lives when compared to their compatriots.

The basics of the Mediterranean Diet include starting every meal with a majority of spices, seeds, legumes, nut, beans, olive oil, vegetables, fruits, and whole grains in moderation. The meal is then added upon with a form of lean protein to match with an emphasis on seafood or fish as a primary component. Keep sugars and dairy-fats to a moderate level. The goal should be to live an overall healthy life, not to follow a strict and limiting set of food-based rules.

When following the Mediterranean diet, your goal should not be to limit total fat consumption, rather it should be to train that focus to be on fats that are healthier in general. This means it is important to stay away from saturated fats as well as oils that are hydrogenated, two things that are known to increase inflammation as well as contribute to heart disease. Wine, in moderation, is also perfectly acceptable as it has been shown to contain numerous healthy side effects as well.

CHAPTER 4

Take Your Diet to the Next Level

When it comes to maximizing the effects of the anti-inflammatory diet, one step that many people find effective is to combine it with the habit of intermittent fasting to supercharge the effectiveness of both. This is due to the fact that intermittent fasting naturally serves to stabilize both glucose and blood sugar levels while naturally decreasing inflammation at the same time. If you do decide to go down this route, however, it is important that you give your body plenty of time to transition to the anti-inflammatory diet first, especially if you previously consumed large amounts of processed foods. After about a month of following the anti-inflammatory diet, you should be ready to add in intermittent fasting as well.

Intermittent fasting is a way of eating to ensure that you get the most out of every meal. The core tenants of intermittent fasting mean that you don't need to change what you are eating, instead, you have to change when you are eating it.

Intermittent fasting is a viable alternative to traditional diets or simply cutting your daily caloric intake which can help fasters lean up without changing the number of calories they consume in a day. In fact, the preferred method of intermittent fasting is to simply eat two large meals every day instead of three (or more) meals in that same period of time.

The body is considered to be in the fed state when it is in the process of absorbing and digesting food. The fed state tends to start roughly five minutes after you begin eating and then lasts for anywhere from three to five hours depending on how long it takes your body to digest the meal. A fed state, in turn, leads to higher levels of insulin which make it much more difficult for the body to burn fat. The period directly after the fed state is referred to as the post-absorptive state which is the period of time where the body is not actively processing food and its insulin levels begin to fall. This state lasts for between eight and twelve hours and directly precedes the fasted state.

The fasted state occurs between nine and twelve hours after the post-absorptive state and is the point where the body's insulin levels are at its lowest, which in turn, make it the period of time where the most fat can be burned during physical activity. Unfortunately, for many people, they rarely go twelve hours without eating which means that no matter how hard they exercise, they are not burning fat as efficiently as possible. However, this also means that you can burn fat and build muscle by simply altering your feeding habits.

Intermittent Fasting Benefits

Building muscle and losing weight are only two of the many benefits that fasting intermittently can lead to. It can also help you to find extra time in a busy schedule as you will find you suddenly don't have to worry about finding time for breakfast every single day. What's more, you will be surprised how much extra money not having to worry about breakfast actually saves you in the long run, even when you factor in the extra amount you are eating for the remaining meals as well. While giving up on breakfast might sound difficult, once new habits begin to form, it will seem like the most natural thing in the world.

Aside from the ancillary benefits, intermittent fasting will also literally help you live longer as being in a prolonged fasting state causes your body to divert extra energy to improving core biological functions as this state sends out emergency signals similar to those that are sent out when your body is starving. A fasting state is quite different from starving, however, and by simply skipping breakfast, you soon won't feel that much hungrier come lunchtime once your body has adapted.

Additional medical benefits include a decrease in the odds of contracting cardiovascular disease and cancer as well as a decreased risk of stroke. It is even known to lessen the aftereffects of chemotherapy. In fact, decreasing your daily calorie count by just 15 percent is known to improve your glucose tolerance and lowers blood pressure, improves oxidative resistance, kidney function, and reproductive effectiveness.

While the reasons behind these benefits aren't entirely clear, it is likely due in part to the fact that intermittent fasting is known to decrease stress while at the same time making your body more resistant to many of the common effects of stress. This is especially true when it comes to organ and digestive tract health. It also improves how your mitochondria work which makes them utilize energy more efficiently and leave you open to less oxidation based damage.

Furthermore, traditional intermittent fasting, as well as alternate-day fasting, are medically approved ways of minimizing the risk of developing type 2 diabetes in those who are already suffering from pre-diabetes. Both of these types of fasting are known to help glucose levels return to normal in as little as 12 months. This benefit can be negated, of course, if the practitioners of intermittent fasting use the fact that they are fasting as an excuse to eat anything and everything during the periods they are not dieting strictly. This is folly, however, as the best way to see long term results is to not treat fasting as something special and to instead think of it as just another part of your daily routine.

To study fasting's astounding efficacy on the human body, an experiment was performed using yeast cells which found that generating an artificial food scarcity for the yeast caused its cells to start dividing slower in response. This literally means that while fasting, each and every one of your cells lives noticeably longer than would be possible with the lack of scarcity.

While there is plenty of real health benefits listed above, what many people ultimately find that they enjoy about intermittent fasting the most is the fact that is just so simple and easy to use. So easy to use, in fact, that studies show that even those who were otherwise considered extremely overweight and had trouble dieting routinely were able to stick with it for 3 months or more, much longer than they were with any other type of more restrictive diet by a power of three or more.

Even better, while on the intermittent diet, these individuals saw just as much average weight loss as anyone else. Perhaps, the best data of all is that a year after the study completed, those who had started with intermittent fasting had managed to lose the most weight overall.

Basics of Fasting

While intermittent fasting isn't that complicated, there are a handful of rules that you are going to want to keep in mind in order to get the most out of the process. It is important to stick with them rigorously in order to see real results in a reasonable period of time.

Burn more calories than you take in: While burning more calories than you consume is a core tenant of many diets, it is crucial when it comes to intermittent fasting as it can be very easy to overeat once you have broken your fast, unintentionally negating all of your hard work. Specifically, you will want to remember that there are 3,500 calories in a pound which means that every week; you are going to need to create this much of a deficit if you hope to lose weight.

While you are likely to lose more than this in the early days of intermittent fasting as your body is still adjusting to the change, 1 pound per week is the average you can expect to lose from any diet in the long term. More than this is unhealthy and can lead to serious negative consequences.

Control yourself: In order to fast effectively, you need to have the self-control to ensure that you can go without eating for at least 12 hours at a time on a regular basis. Any calories consumed during this time will reset the insulin regulation cycle and force your body out of its maximum fat-burning state. Ideally, you will want to

46

consume a calorie deficit of 500 calories per day if you hope to see at least one pound of weight loss per week.

While ensuring that you are not eating too much is going to be important, it is also important to ensure that you remain in control of your habits and don't go out of your way to go longer than is healthy when it comes to fasting. Going too long without eating can cause serious damage to your system as the line between intermittent fasting and starvation is quite thin and it is a line you don't want to cross.

Stick with it: When it comes to using intermittent fasting regularly, it is important to find the variation that works best for you and then settle into a long- term routine as opposed to starting and stopping regularly. While you are sure to see some results right away, it will take about a month for your body to fully adjust to the process which means you need to be committed to the cause and patient. While you are sure to find yourself extremely hungry, at first, after your body has learned when it can start expecting calories, you will find that your hunger more or less returns to normal.

On the other hand, if you rapidly switch between methods of intermittent fasting, or only use it for short bursts now and then, then rather than enhance your body's ability to lose weight naturally while also building muscle, you will instead find it difficult too much of anything effectively as your body will be in a constant state of confusion. If you truly hope to see the types of results you are looking, then the best way to ensure this is the case is to find one schedule of eating that works for you and then stick with it.

Talk to a healthcare professional: While it's true that intermittent fasting helps people to lose weight and build muscle, in addition to a host of other benefits, this doesn't mean it is automatically for everyone or that it doesn't come along with some side effects as well. For starters, when you first transition to an intermittent fasting lifestyle, you are likely to experience diarrhea, constipation, or episodes of both for the first two weeks or so as your body adjusts to its new habits.

Furthermore, it is important to be very careful in not letting yourself binge after you have finished fasting as this can lead to internal damage as well. Regardless of how healthy you plan to be, however, it is important that you talk your plans over with either a dietitian or healthcare professional to ensure you don't end up accidentally doing yourself more harm than good.

Types of Intermittent Fasting

The 16/8 Method: With this method, you are required to fast for 14 to 16 hours each day, and then the remainder of the day, you are technically able to eat whatever you would like. With this eating window, you still have enough time to eat two or three meals without too many issues, so it is still easy to fit this eating schedule into your day without feeling restricted.

This is a really easy method to follow, especially if you pick the right hours to do your fasting. For example, simply stop eating supper at around 8 pm and do not have any late-night snacks. When you get up the next day, you will skip breakfast and start eating around 12 pm. This will put you into a 16-hour fast.

The biggest issue that comes with this option is that some people feel hungry when they wake up in the morning or they have breakfast as part of their morning routine. If you like to eat breakfast, just stop eating around 5 pm and have breakfast at 9 am. You must be careful to not take any late-night snacks in while you are on this plan, but it is much easier compared to some of the other options you may choose.

Studies have shown that both men and women are able to benefit from this method of intermittent fasting. However, it is usually best to go with a little shorter fasting period for women. Women respond well to the daily fast, but they see the best results when they make their fasting window 14 hours instead of 16.

During your fasting window, you are able to have coffee, water, and other non- caloric beverages so that you are not dehydrated. Drinking plenty of water can also be the answer you need to prevent some of those hunger pains.

The 5/2 Method: This is another popular method of intermittent fasting that involves eating regularly for five days during the week while limiting the intake of calories to around 500-600 during the remaining two days. During the two fasting days, the recommended calorie intake for men and women is 600 and 500 calories, respectively. For instance, you can eat regularly on other days, and limit your intake to two small meals amounting to 250 calories each during say Mondays and Thursdays. The two fasting days should be non-consecutive.

The 5:2 diet plan is pretty accommodating and flexible with limited restrictions. You can pick when you want to eat and when you would like to fast depending on a schedule. It is more flexible compared to other methods when it comes to altering fasting and eating times. Some people may enjoy the idea of limiting or controlling their diet only twice a week.

Here comes the big catch now, especially for those who have not fasted before. Going off food for an entire day can be challenging if you are just getting started with intermittent fasting. This is more challenging for people who are required to perform demanding tasks through the day or those with families to look after (preparing meals for children).

Another flip side is that you have to caution against the trap of overeating after fasting for a long duration. Feeling ravenous after fasting for 24 hours may make you overeat; this may not really support your weight loss goals.

Alternate day fasting: With this method, the faster does a partial fast every other day, eating a limited amount of food for one day and then a normal amount the next day, and so on.

Because there are seven days in the week and the diet follows a schedule by the weekday, the dieter uses three specific days of every week to do a partial fast. Dieters using this model commonly choose to diet on Mondays, Wednesdays, and Fridays.

On those days, the dieter consumes only one-fifth of the normal number of calories that he or she consumes on the other days. If you are a man, you likely take in about 2,500 calories per day. If you are a woman, you likely consume about 2,000 calories per day. Therefore, you would consume 500 or 400 calories on Mondays,

Wednesdays, and Fridays, which can easily be done by drinking protein shakes.

Protein shakes are very filling and are also low in calories. High-protein foods and vegetables will also help you to fill up faster. The experts sometimes recommend protein shakes for just the first two weeks of the diet and real food from the third week onward as it is always preferable to anything processed, even if it is marketed as health food.

Working out is not advised on this program if you must work out while on this diet, do a lighter version of your regular workouts on the days that you eat normally.

This diet can effectively drop about 2.5 pounds of weight per week for dieters who cut their calorie intake between 20 and 35 percent, and this is done without the dieter feeling hungry or having to follow a difficult schedule. Additionally, dieting on alternate days never allows leptin levels to fall, which means that the body never stops losing the fat. The dieter must be careful to not binge eat on their off days. This is not a program aimed for beginners or those who only need a slight reduction in weight.

Fat Loss Forever: Fat Loss Forever is an intermittent fasting program that essentially takes the best of all worlds by incorporating ideas from different intermittent fasting programs.

- **Day 1:** Cheat day. A cheat day is exactly what it sounds like. You can eat whatever you want! However, you need to keep what you eat within reason. Eating whatever you want doesn't necessarily mean that you should head straight for the pizza buffet and follow it up with a giant ice cream sundae. Try to keep what you eat within reason. Aim for a high protein intake with a lot of fruits and vegetables. Throw in some special things that you are craving just to make the plan a little bit more fun.

- **Day 2:** Full fast day. Like a cheat day, a full fast day is exactly what it sounds like: you don't consume any calories. You must consume large quantities of water in order to stay hydrated.

- **Day 3:** 16:8 fasting. This day follows a diet schedule that is very similar to lean gains in that you fast for 16 hours and eat for 8.

- **Day 4:** Full fast day. Again, a full fast day is exactly what it sounds like. You won't eat anything.

- **Day 5:** 16:8 fasting. Again, by the end of this day's 16-hour fast, you will have fasted for 36 hours.

- **Day 6:** Warrior diet. On this day, you will follow the procedures that are associated with the warrior diet, as outlined in a previous chapter. You will start off the day with a piece of fruit and a no-carb, high-protein shake, and then fast until 9 pm. As in the warrior diet, you will consume all of the day's calories within a four-hour window. You may want to plan ahead so that this is on a day when you might plan to go out in the evenings. Having something to look forward to and being able to consume a large number of calories in a social setting will make this day's fast easier.

- **Day 7:** Cheat day.

CHAPTER 5

Tips for Success

Have a support system in place: Depending on your relationship with food and your history with dieting, being on a diet can be an extremely stressful time. If you know that sticking to a new diet plan is going to be difficult for you, prepare for this eventuality by ensuring you have a support system in place for when the going gets rough. This could be your friends, family, or even an online community, as long as you have someone to talk to who can tell you to keep it up when the going gets tough, you will find it much easier to avoid running back to old habits for comfort instead.

Additionally, from a practical standpoint, the people in your life are the ones you are going to be eating with most regularly, which means they can act as your willpower when something on the menu looks too tempting. Likewise, even if you don't reach out to these people for help, letting them know that you are on a diet will allow them to refrain from offering you things that are going to tempt your willpower more than you can handle. Being on a diet is nothing to be ashamed about, you will be surprised what sharing your own experiences will draw out of others whom you may have otherwise never expected to be going through the same thing.

Keep yourself from feeling overly hungry: When you are hungry, not just slightly peckish, but extremely famished, it is going to be a lot more difficult for you to think rationally about the situation you are in as your body will be clamoring for you to do something about the situation ASAP. This, in turn, will ultimately make it much more difficult for you to think rationally about your diet goals, potentially putting your long-term plans in jeopardy.

Luckily, it is extremely easy to prevent this scenario from occurring, all you need to do is plan ahead and have something that is diet friendly already lined up to guarantee that you never have to make the choice between the feeling of extreme hunger or sticking to your chosen diet. Additionally, it is important that you make a concentrated effort to never skip meals and always eat at the same time every day to make it easier for your body to know when its next meal is scheduled so it can act accordingly.

Don't completely ignore calories: While following an anti-inflammatory lifestyle means that you don't need to worry about counting calories as much as you would with many other diets, that doesn't mean you should ignore them completely. While an item that is high in healthy fat and contains a medium amount of protein and a small number of carbohydrates might look good on paper, if it also weighs in at 1,000 calories per serving, then you are going to want to give it a wide berth as there is clearly something unhealthy going on somewhere. As such, it is helpful to have a general idea of the number of calories someone of your age, gender, and lifestyle should try and consume in a given day and do your best to stay somewhere within the healthy zone. After all, just because you are going the extra mile to eat in a healthy fashion doesn't mean there is nothing else you can do to be more all-around healthy at all times.

Have the right foods on hand at the right time: If you are exercising regularly, it can be easy to get a little lax now and then when it comes to what you are eating exactly. However, if you use the fact that you exercise as an excuse to eat poorly, you will risk putting your hard work at risk, canceling out all you've done as a result. What's more, you will find that your overall results will be much improved if you make it a point of keeping enough healthy fuel in your system to power your entire workout. Likewise, you are going to want to follow up with an exercise routine with extra protein to ensure your muscles have the tools they need to grow as a result.

Studies show that a longer, milder period of exercise burns the same number of calories as a short, intense workout, while also leaving you less hungry as a result. As such, if you stick to a more moderate workout, you are less likely to feel the need to binge after the fact.

Watch for saturated fats: The key to having a healthy fat consumption is to minimize the consumption of food rich in saturated fats. Although your body needs both kinds of fat, saturated fats from foods derived from plants are enough to provide you with your saturated fat needs. Having high levels of saturated fat in your body leads to heart and cardiovascular disease.

Moreover, it is not enough to replace saturated fat-rich foods with fat-free food products as these are high in carbohydrates and increase the risk of the same disease mentioned. Take a look at the back of a fat-free product and a full-fat product like cream cheese.

Notice that in the fat-free product, there is a lot more sugar than there is in the full-fat one. This is because manufacturers know fat equals flavor. When fat is removed from food, it winds up tasting terrible or is just plain tasteless. They want to make their money, so they add in sugar because they know that consumers love sugar. And what do we know sugar is converted to in your body? That's right, fat! So, you may think you are doing your body good by eating all the fat-free things on the market, but in actuality, you are feeding your body excess sugar which is filling your body up with even more fat.

We know now that saturated fats are not anywhere near as bad as they were once touted to be. It was once feared that a diet heavy in saturated fat would raise cholesterol. Through studies over the years, it has been determined that it is actually a diet rich in carbohydrates that can increase coronary heart disease. This is because a diet high in carbohydrates lowers HDL cholesterol and increases the small particle LDL cholesterol. It is not the saturated fat or the cholesterol from dietary sources that raise the level of the small bad LDL cholesterol; it is the consumption of too many carbohydrates. Saturated fat is actually great for your liver, your brain, your heart, your nervous system, and more.

Spice it up: If you find yourself feeling hungry at the end of a meal, and then making less than optimal choices when you feel the need to snack, it might not be your macros that are out of whack. Rather, you may be light on the spice that can help tell your body that you are full. Capsaicin, one of the most common ways of making foods spicy, is also known to increase the rate at which endorphins are released into the body. Not only do endorphins make you happy, but they also leave you feeling fuller as a result.

Make a point of taking in more iron: During the 14-day meal plan, you are going to want to keep your metabolism at the highest rate possible, and eating plenty of foods that are rich in iron is a big part of that. The fact of the matter is if your body doesn't have the iron it needs to keep the cells of the body full of oxygen, then it will slow down your metabolism until it can find more. Don't limit your body's potential, ensure you are well-stocked on iron.

Leave the serving dish where you can't see it: While it may be hard to believe, the truth of the matter is that much of the hunger you feel come mealtime is psychological. What this means is that if you feel the need to go back for a second helping, this is often because the food is already there and readily available. This means that out of sight out of mind works on your appetite as well as anything else. Do yourself a favor and leave the extra servings far from where you are actually consuming the food and you should find that you are less inclined to get up and get a second serving. This will also give your food the time it needs to make it to your intestines so that you don't feel the need to keep eating when you are actually already full.

Set aside time to cook: Eating out regularly while following the anti- inflammatory diet can be a tricky subject at best. What's worse, trying to find processed "healthy" options will only lead to unhealthy choices that might also compromise your diet. As such, it is important to always be prepared with your own healthy snacks as well as making sure to set aside the time you need to make breakfast, lunch, and dinner every day. Start by cooking extra portions and freezing them for later meals during particularly busy days and really get into the habit of cooking by doing it for every single meal. Give it some time and cooking each meal will begin to feel natural and fun.

Stock up on necessities: While it is true that many healthy items are more expensive than comparable amounts of less healthy foods, a lot of the items you will be eating can be purchased in bulk for prices comparable to those of lesser items. Plan out your meals for two weeks or more and head to your local bulk supplier and you will be surprised at the deals you can find. After all, many of the items you will be purchasing have quite a long shelf-life. Take advantage of that fact.

Take in fewer calories than you expend: While the modern weight loss industry would have you believe otherwise, the truth of the matter is that losing weight is as simple as eating fewer calories than you expend each day in energy. If you do 500 calories a day, then you will lose a pound of fat each week which is equal to 3,500 calories. This won't necessarily mean you will be a pound lighter, however, because you may have to account for added muscle in the equation as well. Nevertheless, what you want to do is burn fat anyway, so this is a good place to start. As such, it is important to take the meal plan as an outline and tailor the caloric intake to your specific lifestyle, goals, and personal details. What's more, if you aren't already exercising every day, you will find that your results are going to be a lot more positive if you start.

Drink more green tea: Studies show that as little as three cups of green tea per day is enough to cause nearly a 5 percent bump to your metabolism. While this might not seem like much on the surface, it is akin to about 60 extra calories burned per day. This means that you will burn an extra pound every 60 days, and help reduce your risk of cancer in the bargain. While this might not seem like much, when compounded against the other tips outlined below, it is nothing to sneeze at.

Substitutions: When you first begin transitioning to a healthier lifestyle, you may find that you routinely get cravings for specific types of foods that are now off of the table. One of the biggest reasons that many people fail to start a new diet once they have committed to it is they don't account for just how addictive many types of processed foods really are. Don't fall victim to the lure of unhealthy options, have a plan in place by keeping the following list in mind. The next time you get a craving, consider countering it in the following ways.

- Replace chocolate ice cream with chocolate flavored fat-free Greek yogurt.

- Replace an ice cream sundae with frozen yogurt topped with fruit.

- Replace cheese doodles with non-processed cubes of actual cheese for a snack full of healthy fats.

- Replace chips and dip with vegetables and hummus.

- Replace a candy bar with a healthy protein bar.

- Replace potato chips with a small amount of air-popped popcorn.

- Replace a cheeseburger with soy or black bean patty.

- Replace other salty favorites with healthy nut options instead.

Once you are ready to get started, it is important to do yourself a favor for later and take a number of "before" photographs and measurements to aid yourself in committing long term by proving yourself the opportunity to look back on how far you have come. This means you will want to weigh yourself on a scale as well as determine your current level of muscle mass and body fat. Don't forget to measure your shoulders, chest, waist, calves, thighs, and arms for the best results.

While it may be difficult to look at yourself in such an analytical light now, you will be happy in a few weeks' time when you have a baseline to compare your progress to. Write down your current measurements and put them someplace you will see them every morning. Write down the new ones each time you take them and keep them in the same place. This visual representation of the timeline will make transitioning to the new lifestyle successfully much more manageable.

Don't forget to take the stress and sleep patterns into account: When it comes to weight loss, there is only so much that improving your diet and exercise habits can do. The rest has to come from improving your habits. Stress that sticks around long enough to be considered chronic is known to regularly make you hungrier than normal, which typically leads to weight gain. This isn't just a mindset thing either; studies show that this type of chronic stress alters the balance of the hormones in your system, leading to the increased feelings of hunger.

In addition to striving to remain as stress-free as possible, it is important to make a concentrated effort to go to bed at the same time every night and to wake up without the aid of an alarm whenever possible. Getting in sync with your circadian rhythms won't just make you feel better; it will cause your hormone levels to rebalance themselves while also improving your digestion.

CHAPTER 6

14-Day Meal Plan

Day 1

Breakfast: Black Bean, Spinach, Mushroom, and Tomato Quiche

Makes enough for: 4

Time required for proper preparation: 30 minutes

Suggested cooking time: 50 minutes

Time total: 80 minutes

What to Use - Crust

- Water (1.5 T + 3 T)

- Olive oil (1 T)

- Salt (.5 tsp.)

- Oregano (1 tsp.)

- Parsley (1 tsp.)

- Buckwheat flour (1 c)

- Almond flour (1 c)

- Flax (1 T, ground)

What to Use - Quiche

- Black beans (14 oz.)
- Olive oil (1 T)
- Yellow onion (1 sliced)
- Leek (1 sliced)
- Garlic (3 cloves minced)
- Cremini mushrooms (3 c sliced)
- Chives (.5 c chopped)
- Basil leaves (.5 c chopped)
- Tomatoes (.3 c chopped)
- Baby spinach (1 c)
- Yeast (2 T)
- Oregano (1 tsp.)
- Sea salt (1 tsp.)
- Pepper (as desired)
- Red pepper flakes (as desired)

What to Do

- Ensure that your oven has been preheated to 350°F.
- Coat a tart pan or glass cooking dish with cooking spray.

- Combine the water and flax together and leave it to thicken.

- Combine the salt, oregano, parsley, buckwheat flour, oat flour, and almond flour together in a large bowl.

- Mix in the flax before adding the water and mixing until it gains the consistency of cookie dough.

- Add the dough to the greased dish and form a crust. Add a few holes to allow air to vent properly.

- Place the dish in the oven and bake for 15 minutes.

- Remove dish and turn the oven to 375°F.

- Add the beans to food processor until smooth; a splash of almond milk improves this process.

- Coat a pan in olive oil and place it on the stove above a burner that has been turned to medium heat.

- Add in the onion, the leek, and the garlic and let them cook for 2 minutes before mixing in the salt and mushrooms and letting them cook for 10 minutes.

- Mix in the red pepper flakes, pepper, salt, oregano, yeast, spinach, tomatoes, and herbs and let everything cook until the spinach wilts.

- Remove the pan from the stove and add in the beans before mixing well.

- Add the mixture to the crust and let it bake for 35 minutes.

- Let it cool for 20 minutes prior to serving.

Lunch: Beef Stew

Makes enough for: 8

Time required for proper preparation: 15 minutes

Suggested cooking time: 8 hours

Time total: 8 hours and 15 minutes

What to Use

- Apple cider vinegar (2 T)
- Water (1.5 c)
- Apple cider (2 c)
- Apples (1 c peeled)
- Celery (.5 c)
- Onion (1 c)
- Carrots (1.5 c)
- Coconut oil (3 T)
- Thyme (.25 tsp.)
- Black pepper (.25 tsp.)
- White flour (7 T)
- Beef cubes (2 lbs.)
- Potatoes (1.5 c)

What to Do

- Prepare potatoes by removing excess potassium if required.

- In a small bowl, mix together the thyme, black pepper, and flour before coating the beef in the results.

- Add the oil to a skillet before placing the skillet on the stove over a burner turned to medium heat before adding in the beef and letting it brown.

- Remove the meat from the skillet before slicing the celery, onion, carrots, and apple.

- Add the carrots to a slow cooker, then the potatoes, followed by the onions, then the celery, the beef and top it all off with the apple.

- Combine the water and vinegar before adding them to the slow cooker and letting it cook on low heat for 8 hours.

- Prior to eating, turn the heat to high, combine 0.5 c of water and 4 T of flour and add them to the slow cooker and mix well.

- Serve hot and enjoy.

Snack: Wings with Teriyaki Sauce

This recipe makes 12 servings and requires about 5 hours of preparation

Makes enough for: 12

Time required for proper preparation: 4 hours

Suggested cooking time: 30 minutes

Time total: 4 hours and 30 minutes

What to Use

- Ginger (.5 tsp. ground)

- Balsamic vinegar (.3 c)

- Garlic powder (.5 tsp.)

- Brown sugar (.25 c)

- Teriyaki sauce (2 T reduced-sodium)

- Black pepper (.25 tsp.)

- Water (.5 c)

- Chicken wings (24)

- Soy sauce (2 T reduced-sodium)

What to Do

- Add the chicken wings to a large container with a lid.

- Mix the ginger, balsamic vinegar, garlic powder, brown sugar, teriyaki sauce, soy sauce, black pepper, and water together in a small bowl before adding the results to the container as well before placing the container in the refrigerator to allow the wings to marinate for at least 4 hours.

- Ensure your oven is heated to 400°F.

- Add the wings to a baking dish before adding the dish to the oven and letting them cook for 30 minutes.

- Serve hot and enjoy.

Dinner: Shepherd's Pie

Makes enough for: 4

Time required for proper preparation: 30 minutes

Suggested cooking time: 60 minutes

Time total: 90 minutes

What to Use

- Soy cheese (.5 c shredded)

- Soy beef (14 oz.)

- Pepper (as desired)

- Garlic (1 clove minced)

- Italian seasoning (1 tsp.)

- Tomato (1 chopped)

- Celery (3 stalks chopped)

- Carrots (2 chopped)

- Yellow onion (1 chopped)

- Vegetable oil (1 T)

- Salt (2 tsp)

- Vegan cream cheese (3 T)

- Olive oil (.25 c)

- Soy milk (.5 c)

- Mayonnaise (.5 c vegan)

- Potatoes (5 cubed)

- Peas (.5 c)

What to Do

- Ensure your oven is preheated to 400°F.

- Using baking spray, coat a baking dish.

- Add the potatoes to a pot before covering them in cold water. Add the pot to a burner turned to a high/medium heat and let it boil. Reduce the heat to low/medium and then continue boiling the potatoes for 25 minutes.

- Add in the salt, vegan cream cheese, olive oil, soy milk, and vegan mayonnaise before mashing potatoes.

- Coat a pan in the oil and place it on the stove above a burner that has been turned to medium heat.

- Add in the tomato, peas, celery, carrots, and onion and let them cook for about 10 minutes before mixing in the pepper, garlic, and Italian seasoning.

- Turn the heat to low/medium before adding in the soy ground beef and let it cook for 5 minutes.

- Add the mixture in the skillet to the baking dish before adding the potatoes on top and then covering it all with the vegan cheese substitute.

- Add the baking dish to the oven and let it cook for roughly 20 minutes.

- Serve hot and enjoy.

Dessert: Saffron Panna Cotta

Makes enough for: 4

Time required for proper preparation: 2 hours

Suggested cooking time: 0 minutes

Time total: 2 hours

What to Use

- Raspberries (12)

- Almonds (1 T chopped)

- Honey (1 T)

- Saffron (1 pinch)

- Vanilla (.25 tsp)

- Whipping cream (2 c)

- Water (as desired)

- Unflavored gelatin (.5 T)

What to Do

- Follow the instructions on your gelatin and mix in some water. Set to the side to let it bloom.

- Place honey, saffron, vanilla, and cream to a pot and let it boil. Turn the heat down and allow it to simmer.

- Take the pan off the stove and mix in the gelatin until it is completely dissolved.

- Add the mixture to six ramekins. Top with plastic wrap and refrigerate for two hours at least. Toast the almonds and serve the pannacotta with the nuts and berries.

DAY 2

Breakfast: Breakfast Frittata

Makes enough for: 4

Time required for proper preparation: 5 minutes

Suggested cooking time: 2 hours

Time total: 2 hours and 5 minutes

What to Use

- Black pepper (as desired)

- Salt (as desired)

- Egg (8 beaten)

- Red onion (.25 c diced)

- Red bell pepper (1.5 c diced)

- Spinach (.75 c)

What to Do

- Coat your slow cooker with cooking spray before adding in the salt, black pepper, eggs, red onions, red pepper, and spinach. Cover the slow cooker and let it cook for 2 hours on low heat.

- Freeze the remainder in Ziploc bags and reheat them for 45 seconds in the microwave on the high setting.

Lunch: Grilled Peach and Shrimp Salad

Makes enough for: 4

Time required for proper preparation: 15 minutes

Suggested cooking time: 15 minutes

Time total: 30 minutes

What to Use - Pesto

- Black pepper (as needed)

- Salt (as needed)

- Lemon juice (2 tsp.)

- Coconut oil (.5 c)

- Garlic (2 cloves minced)

- Basil (1.5 c torn)

- Pistachios (1 c unsalted)

What to Use - Salad

- Pistachios (.3 c unsalted)

- Cherry tomatoes (1 c halved)

- Cucumber (1 sliced)

- Mixed greens (5 c)

- Peaches (3 chopped in half, pits removed)

- Garlic powder (as desired)

- Salt (as desired)

- Shrimp (1 lb. deveined, peeled)

- Coconut oil (2 T divided, melted)

What to Use - Dressing

- Black pepper (as desired)

- Salt (1 pinch)

- Dijon mustard (1 T)

- Raw honey (1 T)

- Lemon juice (.25 c)

- Olive oil (.5 c)

What to Do - Shrimp

- In a food processor, add in the pistachios and pulse well before adding in the cloves of garlic as well as the basil. Process again before adding in the coconut oil while pulsing until the pesto reaches the desired thickness before mixing in the lemon juice.

- Add the oil to a pan before adding the pan to the stove on top of a burner turned to medium heat. Add in half of the ghee before adding in the shrimp and seasoning as desired.

- Let the shrimp cook in the pan for 60 seconds per side before adding in 2 T pesto and coating well.

What to Do - Salad

- Add a pan for grilling to a burner set to medium heat before greasing the peaches with the remaining ghee and grilling each peach for 1.5 minutes per side.

- Combine all of the salad ingredients together as desired.

- Combine all of the dressing ingredients in a jar and shake well before topping the salad.

Snack: Carrot Soup with Coriander

This recipe takes about 5 minutes to prepare, 40 minutes to cook, and makes 4 servings.

Makes enough for: 4

Time required for proper preparation: 5 minutes

Suggested cooking time: 40 minutes

Time total: 45 minutes

What to Use

- Vegetable stock (2 pints)

- Garlic (2 cloves)

- Coriander (1 tsp. ground)

- Onion (1 peeled)

- Carrots (450 grams chopped, peeled)

What to Do

- Prepare the onion for sautéing before adding in the garlic after it has been crushed.

- Mix in the chopped carrots and let them cook for 5 minutes.

- Add in the coriander and the vegetable stock.

- Let the results simmer until the carrot has become soft; this should take approximately 30 minutes.

- Place the contents of the pan into a blender and puree.

- Add coriander as desired and serve.

Dinner: Lamb Burger

Makes enough for: 4

Time required for proper preparation: 15 minutes

Suggested cooking time: 10 minutes

Time total: 25 minutes

What to Use

- Arugula (8 leaves)

- Feta cheese (8 oz. sliced)

- Ciabatta rolls (4 sliced)

- Green tomato (1 sliced)

- Sweet onion (1 sliced)

- Salt (.5 tsp.)

- Garlic (1 clove minced)

- Lemon zest (1 lemon)

- Plain Greek Yogurt (16 oz.)

- Pepper (.5 tsp.)

- Salt (1 tsp.)

- Garlic (1 tsp. minced)

- Ginger root (1 tsp. minced)

- Mint (3 T chopped)

- Lamb (1 lb. ground)

- Turkey (.5 lbs. ground)

What to Do

- Add oil to your grill and heat it to a high/medium heat.

- In a large bowl, combine the pepper, tsp. salt, tsp. garlic, ginger, mint, turkey, and lamb together.

- Portion out patties.

- In a small bowl, combine the remaining salt, garlic, lemon zest, and Greek yogurt together and place in the refrigerator.

- Place the patties on the grill and let them cook for 3 minutes on either side.

- Add the buns to the grill and let each side cook for 60 seconds, grill vegetables as desired.

- Combine ingredients, serve hot and enjoy.

Dessert: Spice Cake

This recipe needs 15 minutes to prepare, 15 minutes to cook and will make 12 cupcakes.

Makes enough for: 12

Time required for proper preparation: 15 minutes

Suggested cooking time: 15 minutes

Time total: 30 minutes

What to Use - Frosting

- Lemon zest (.5 lemons)

- Vanilla extract (1 tsp.)

- Erythritol (3 T)

- Coconut oil (2 T)

- Cream cheese (8 oz.)

What to Use - Cake

- Clove (.25 tsp. ground)

- Ginger (.5 tsp.)

- Allspice (.5 tsp.)

- Nutmeg (.5 tsp.)

- Cinnamon (.5 tsp.)

- Vanilla extract (1 tsp.)

- Baking powder (2 tsp.)

- Eggs (4 large)

- Water (5 T)

- Butter (.5 c)

- Erythritol (.75 c)

- Almond flour (2 c)

What to Do

- Start by making sure your oven is heated to 350°F.

- Combine the erythritol and the coconut oil in a mixing bowl and mix until smooth.

- Add in a pair of the eggs and combine thoroughly before repeating the process with the remaining eggs.

- Mix the ground clove, ginger, allspice, nutmeg, cinnamon, and vanilla extract together in a small bowl before adding the results to the batter and mixing well before finally adding in the water.

- Grease a cupcake tin before adding in the batter, taking special care to leave room for the batter to rise.

- Place the cupcake tin in the oven and let the cupcakes bake 15 minutes.

- As the cupcakes are baking, mix together the lemon zest, vanilla, erythritol, coconut oil, and cream cheese in a mixing bowl and mix well.

- After taking the cupcakes out of the oven, let them sit for 15 minutes prior to frosting.

DAY 3

Breakfast: Cacao Cereal

Makes enough for: 1

Time required for proper preparation: 30 minutes

Suggested cooking time: 30 minutes

Time total: 60 minutes

What to Use

- Chia Seeds (0.5 c)

- Hemp Hearts (4 T)

- Coconut Oil (2 T)

- Raw Cacao Nibs (2 T)

- Organic Sugar-Free Vanilla Extract (1 T)

- Swerve (1 T)

- Fine Psyllium Powder (1 T)

- Water (1 c)

What to Do

- Ensure your oven is preheated to 285°F.

- In a large mixing bowl, cover chia seeds with water, stir once and let sit.

- After 5 minutes, add fine psyllium powder, swerve, vanilla extract, coconut oil, and hemp hearts into the bowl with chia seeds. Blend until ingredients are thoroughly mixed and chia seeds start to gel.

- Add cacao nibs to a bowl and stir them into the dough.

- Place two large pieces of wax paper down. Turn dough out onto wax paper and roll until dough is about 11 x 14 inches across.

- Take hands to roll dough into cylinder and place on parchment paper with the shiny side up.

- Flatten dough with fingers before you place another piece of parchment paper over it. Flatten until it is .25 inches thick.

- Bake for 15 minutes. The dough should dry significantly and be almost completely dry after 15 minutes.

- Remove the cookie sheet and carefully flip dough over, removing the parchment paper that will now be on the top side. Cook for an additional 15-25 minutes until dough is completely dry. Check frequently after 15 minutes to ensure cereal doesn't burn.

- Remove cereal from oven and let cool to at least room temperature before breaking up into smaller chunks to eat with cream or coconut milk. The remainder can successfully be stored someplace air-tight for as long as 3 days.

Lunch: Keto Tuna Melt

Makes enough for: 1

Time required for proper preparation: 5 minutes

Suggested cooking time: 15 minutes

Time total: 20 minutes

What to Use - Bread

- Baking powder (.5 tsp.)

- Psyllium husk (.5 T powder)

- Salt (1 pinch)

- Cream cheese (4 oz.)

- Eggs (3)

What to Use - Filling

- Cheese (shredded 4 oz.)

- Garlic (.5 cloves minced)

- Lemon juice (.5 tsp.)

- Olive oil (1 can)

- Dill pickles (.25 c chopped)

- Celery (1 stalk)

- Sour cream (.3 c)

What to Do - Bread

- Start by making sure your oven is heated to 300°F.

- Separate the eggs from their yolks and save both in separate bowls.

- Add salt to the whites and whisk well.

- Add the cream cheese to the yolks and mix well before adding in the baking powder and psyllium.

- Combine the two bowls and mix well before adding the results to a baking sheet so that it will form eight slices.

- Bake in the center of the oven for 25 minutes

What to Do - Filling

- Start by making sure your oven is heated to 350°F.

- Combine all of the filling ingredients, minus the cheese, together in a bowl and mix well.

- Place two slices of bread onto a lined baking sheet and top with filling and finish with cheese.

- Bake for 15 minutes.

Snack: Veggie Quiche

Makes enough for: 2

Time required for proper preparation: 10 minutes

Suggested cooking time: 40 minutes

Time total: 50 minutes

What to Use

- Basil (2 T chopped)

- Coconut milk (3 fluid oz.)

- Eggs (4)

- Ground black pepper (as desired)

- Thyme leaves (2 tsp.)

- Spinach (16 oz.) chopped)

- Asparagus (4.5 oz. sliced)

- Shitake mushrooms (2.5 o. sliced)

- Extra virgin olive oil (1 T)

- Leeks (2 sliced thin)

What to Do

- Ensure your oven is heated to 350°F.

- Add the oil to a pan before placing it over a burner turned to a high/medium heat.

- Add in the mushrooms and leeks and let them sauté for 5 minutes.

- Mix in the asparagus and let it cook for an additional 4 minutes before mixing in the thyme and spinach and letting everything cook until the spinach starts to wilt.

- Once this happens, remove the pan from the burner before seasoning as desired and letting the pan cool.

- Combine the coconut milk and eggs together in a mixing bowl before adding in the vegetable mixture and mixing well.

- Add the results to a pie tin and place the tin in the oven to cook for 30 minutes.

- Top with basil and then let the quiche cool for 5 minutes prior to cutting and serving.

Dinner: Stir Fry with Cabbage

Makes enough for: 4

Time required for proper preparation: 15 minutes

Suggested cooking time: 30 minutes

Time total: 45 minutes

What to Use

- Wasabi paste (.5 T)

- Low-carb mayonnaise (1 c)

- Sesame oil (1 T)

- Ginger (1 T grated)

- Chili flakes (1 tsp.)

- Scallions (3 sliced)

- Garlic (2 cloves)

- White wine vinegar (1 T)

- Black pepper (.25 tsp. ground)

- Onion powder (1 tsp.)

- Salt (1 tsp.)

- Beef (1.3 lbs. ground)

- Coconut oil (4 T)

- Cabbage (1.6 lbs. shredded)

What to Do

- Add 4 T to a frying pan before placing the pan on a burner set to a high/medium heat.

- Add the cabbage to the frying pan and let it cook, taking care to prevent it from browning. Season using vinegar and spices before continuing to stir and fry an additional 2 minutes before removing the cabbage from heat.

- Add the remainder of the coconut oil to the frying pan before adding in the ginger, chili flakes, and garlic and sautéing for 3 minutes.

- Add in the meat and let it brown before reducing the heat to medium and adding in the cabbage and scallions. Season using pepper, salt, and sesame oil and ensure everything is hot prior to serving.

- Combine the wasabi paste and the mayo and add the results to the stir fry prior to serving.

Dessert: Banana Strawberry Parfait

Makes enough for: 1

Time required for proper preparation: 5 minutes

Suggested cooking time: 10 minutes

Time total: 15 minutes

What to Use

- Strawberry Greek Yogurt (6 oz.)

- Banana (1 sliced)

- Quinoa (1 c)

- Water (1 c)

What to Do

- Combine the quinoa and the water together in a pot before placing it on top of a burner set to high heat and letting it boil. Once it has, let the quinoa simmer until it has absorbed all of the water. You will see small holes throughout the quinoa. Fluff with a fork and allow to cool.

- Mix in the banana and yogurt prior to serving.

DAY 4

Breakfast: Chickpea Omelet with Spinach

Makes enough for: 8

Time required for proper preparation: 5 minutes

Suggested cooking time: 15 minutes

Time total: 20 minutes

What to Use

- Salt (as desired)

- Black pepper (as desired)

- Chickpea flour (.5 c)

- Flax meal (3 T)

- Turmeric (2 tsp.)

- Garlic powder (1 tsp.)

- Spinach (4 c chopped)

What to Do

- In a large bowl, combine the spinach, garlic powder, turmeric, flax meal, pepper, salt, and chickpea flour together and mix well.

- Add a sauté pan to the stove over a burner turned to medium heat.

- Add .3 c of water to the bowl of dry ingredients before whisking as needed to ensure an even consistency.

- Add in the spinach or other vegetables and mix well before adding the results to the sauté pan.

- Let the omelet cook until it begins to bubble before flipping it and repeating the process.

- Serve hot and enjoy.

Lunch: Sesame and Ginger Quinoa Salad

Makes enough for: 4

Time required for proper preparation: 10 minutes

Suggested cooking time: 15 minutes

Time total: 25 minutes

What to Use

- Water (2 c)
- Edamame (1.5 c)
- Quinoa (1 c rinsed)
- Salt (.25 tsp)
- Carrots (3 medium diced)
- Chili (.5 diced)
- Yellow pepper (.5 diced)
- Sesame oil (2 T)
- Rice vinegar (2 T)
- Red cabbage (1 c chopped)
- Sesame seeds (1 T)
- Ginger (.4 tsp)

What to Do

- Turn a boiler to high heat before combining the water, quinoa, and salt together in a covered pot and placing the pot on the boiler. After it reaches the boiling point, reduce the heat to low and let the quinoa cook for 15 minutes or until the water is completely absorbed.

- Combine the peppers, carrots, cabbage, edamame, and the quinoa in a bowl and mix well.

- Separately, in another bowl, combine the ginger, sesame oil, rice vinegar, and sesame seeds together and mix well.

- Combine the two bowls prior to serving.

Snack: Herb Dip with Feta

Makes enough for: 5

Time required for proper preparation: 35 minutes

Suggested cooking time: 15 minutes

Time total: 50 minutes

What to Use

- Extra virgin olive oil (1 T chopped)

- Chives (.25 c chopped)

- Mint (.25 c fresh, chopped)

- Dill (.25 c, fresh, chopped)

- Parsley (.25 c fresh, chopped)

- Ground pepper (1 tsp.)

- Garlic salt (1 tsp.)

- Lemon juice (1 T)

- Feta cheese (.5 c crumbled)

- Low fat plain Greek yogurt (.75 c)

- White beans (15 oz. rinsed)

What to Do

- In a food processor, combine the pepper, garlic, salt, lemon juice, feta, Greek yogurt, and beans. Process until smooth.

- Add in the chives, mint, dill, and parsley and process as desired.

- Chill prior to serving.

Dinner: Stir Fry with Chickpeas and Quinoa

Makes enough for: 6

Time required for proper preparation: 10 minutes

Suggested cooking time: 10 minutes

Time total: 20 minutes

What to Use

- Black pepper (as desired)
- Kosher salt (as desired)
- Spinach leaves (4 c packed loose)
- Tomatoes (3 diced)
- Chickpeas (3 c cooked)
- Quinoa (4 c cooked)
- Red chili (sliced, seeded)
- Ginger (1 inch chopped)
- Garlic (4 cloves chopped)
- Red bell pepper (1 sliced thin)
- Onion (1 sliced thin)
- Red pepper flakes (.25 tsp.)
- Curry powder (2 tsp.)

- Garam masala (2 tsp.)

- Cumin (2 tsp. ground)

- Paprika (1.5 tsp.)

- Chili powder (2 tsp.)

- Coconut oil (3 T)

What to Do

- Place the coconut oil into a cooking pot before placing the pot on the stove on top of a burner set to a medium/low heat. Add in the chili powder, smoked paprika, cumin, red curry powder, and garam masala and let them simmer for two minutes.

- Add in the garlic as well as the onion before turning the heat to medium. Stir for 3 minutes before adding in the ginger and the pepper slices. Let the pepper slices cook for 60 seconds before adding in the quinoa and cooking another 60 seconds.

- Mix in the chickpeas and let them cook 2 minutes, stirring regularly before adding in the spinach as well as the tomatoes and letting everything cook 3 additional minutes.

Dessert: Blueberry Dessert Bars

Makes enough for: 15

Time required for proper preparation: 15 minutes

Suggested cooking time: 45 minutes

Time total: 60 minutes

What to Use

- White sugar (1 c +.5 c)

- Salt (.25 tsp)

- Cornstarch (3 tsp)

- Blueberries (4 c fresh)

- Cinnamon (as desired)

- Egg (1)

- Shortening (1 c)

- All-purpose flour (3 c)

- Baking powder (1 tsp)

What to Do

- Ensure your oven is set to 375°F.

- Prepare a baking pan (9 x 13 in.) for use by greasing it.

- Combine the baking powder, 3 c flour, and 1 c sugar together in a mixing bowl and combine thoroughly. Add in the cinnamon and salt before using a fork to blend in the egg and shortening. The resulting dough should be crumbly.

- Add half of the dough to the baking pan and press it down firmly to form a crust.

- In a separate bowl, mix together the remaining sugar and the cornstarch before adding in the blueberries and mixing well. Add the results to the pan before topping with the rest of the dough.

- Place the baking pan in the oven for 45 minutes or until you can successfully push a toothpick through the middle of the pan and pull it out clean.

- Allow the pan to cool completely before cutting into squares.

Day 5

Breakfast: Granola with Peanut Butter

Makes enough for: 34

Time required for proper preparation: 5 minutes

Suggested cooking time: 2 hours

Time total: 125 minutes

What to Use

- Cinnamon (.5 tsp.)

- Maple syrup (.25 c)

- Water (6 T)

- Coconut oil (6 T)

- Brown sugar (.5 c)

- Peanut butter (1 c)

- Peanuts (.5 c)

- Sunflower seeds (.5 c)

- Coconut (.5 shredded)

- Wheat germ (.5 c)

- Rolled oats (6 c)

What to Do

- Add the peanuts, sunflower seeds, coconut, wheat germ, and rolled oats to a slow cooker.

- Add the cinnamon, maple syrup, water, oil, brown sugar, and peanut butter to a saucepan and mix well before placing it on the stove over a burner turned to medium heat and continue to stir while everything melts.

- Add the results to the slow cooker and ensure everything is well coated.

- Leave the lid of the slow cooker slightly ajar and turn the slow cooker to low heat for about 2 hours, stirring regularly. Granola is ready when it is golden brown.

- Remove the granola from the slow cooker and spread it on a cookie sheet to cool completely before moving to an airtight container.

Lunch: Mushroom Stew

Makes enough for: 4

Time required for proper preparation: 10 minutes

Suggested cooking time: 15 minutes

Time total: 25 minutes

What to Use

- Chopped canned tomatoes (28 oz.)
- Dried oregano (.25 tsp.)
- Pepper
- Salt
- Minced garlic cloves (5)
- Chopped carrot (.5 c)
- Chopped celery (.5 c)
- Chopped red onion (.5 c)
- Veggie stock (1.25 c)
- Grated ginger (1 T)
- Chopped white mushrooms (4 oz.)
- Chopped shiitake mushrooms (8 oz.)
- Chopped basil leaves (.25 c)

- Turmeric powder (1.5 tsp.)

What to Do

- Turn on the Instant Pot and add in .25 c of stock. When the stock is warm, add in the garlic, ginger, carrot, celery, onion, and both mushrooms.

- Cook those ingredients for five minutes. Then add in the rest of your stock along with the oregano, turmeric, pepper, salt, and tomatoes.

- Cover the Instant Pot and cook on a High setting for 10 minutes. Divide the finished mixture up and enjoy.

Snack: Stir Fried Vegetables

Makes enough for: 4

Time required for proper preparation: 5 minutes

Suggested cooking time: 7 minutes

Time total: 12 minutes

What to Use

- Water chestnuts (.25 c drained)

- Bamboo shoots (.25 c drained)

- Carrot (.5 sliced thin)

- Snow peas (1 c)

- Red bell pepper (1 in. squares)

- Bok choy (2 c chopped)

- Ginger (1.5 tsp. minced, peeled)

- Garlic cloves (2 minced)

- Low-sodium soy sauce (1 T)

- Chicken broth (.25 c)

What to Do

- Mix together the ginger, garlic, soy sauce, and chicken broth.

- Add the oil to a skillet before placing it on the stove over a burner turned to a high/medium heat. Add in the bell pepper and bok choy and let them cook for 3 minutes before adding in the carrot and snow peas. Reduce the heat and allow everything to cook, stirring regularly until the sauce is thick and the veggies are crisp.

- Add in the water chestnuts and bamboo shoots and let them heat for about a minute prior to serving.

Dinner: Spicy Chicken and Beans

Makes enough for: 4

Time required for proper preparation: 10 minutes

Suggested cooking time: 10 minutes

Time total: 20 minutes

What to Use

- Black pepper (as desired)

- Sea salt (as desired)

- Mexican cheese blend (.25 c)

- Chunky salsa (.5 c)

- Corn (1 c frozen)

- Black beans (15 oz. drained, rinsed)

- Coconut oil (1 T)

- Chicken breasts 4 oz. (4)

- Chipotle seasoning (3 tsp.)

What to Do

- Coat the chicken in the Mrs. Dash.

- Add the oil to a skillet before placing it on the stove over a burner turned to medium heat before adding in the chicken and letting it cook for about 4 minutes per side or until it reaches an internal temperature of 165°F.

- Remove the chicken from the skillet and add in the salsa, corn, and beans and let them warm for about 3 minutes.

- Top the chicken with the cheese and allow it to melt.

- Serve .5 c of beans with each chicken breast.

Dessert: Macaroons

Makes enough for: 10

Time required for proper preparation: 10 minutes

Suggested cooking time: 15 minutes

Time total: 25 minutes

What to Use

- Egg whites (3)

- Coconut oil (1 T)

- Vanilla extract 91 T)

- Swerve (2 T)

- Coconut (.5 c shredded)

- Almond flour (.25 c)

What to Do

- Start by making sure your oven is heated to 400°F.

- Combine the swerve, coconut, and almond flour in a mixing bowl and mix well.

- Add the coconut oil to a small saucepan before placing it on top of a burner turned to medium heat. After the oil melts, add in the vanilla extra and mix well.

- Place a medium-sized mixing bowl in the freezer to aid in the mounting of the egg whites.

- Once the bowl is chilled, add in the egg whites and whisk until they become stiff. At this point, you will add them into the flour mix gently, to ensure that you do not overmix and retain as much egg white volume as possible.

- Add the results to a cookie sheet so it makes 10 portions.

- Place the baking sheet in the oven for 8 minutes and the macaroons have browned on top.

- Let cool prior to removing from the baking sheet.

DAY 6

Breakfast: Bok Choy and Avocado Smoothie

Makes enough for: 1

Time required for proper preparation: 5 minutes

Suggested cooking time: 0 minutes

Time total: 5 minutes

What to Use

- Ice cubes (6)

- Your choice of sweetener (as desired)

- Avocado (.5 medium)

- Plain whey protein powder (1 scoop)

- Coconut oil (2 T)

- Bok choy (2 oz.)

- Pear (.5 chopped)

- Chia seeds (2 T)

- Rishi mushroom (1 T)

What to Do

- Slice the avocado lengthwise before removing the seeds and the skin. Add the sliced avocado, along with the remaining ingredients to your blender.

- Add all of the ingredients, save the ice cubes, to the blender and blend on low speed until pureed. Thin with water as needed.

- Add in the ice cubes and blend until the smoothie reaches your desired consistency.

Lunch: Feta and Spinach Bake

Makes enough for: 6

Time required for proper preparation: 10 minutes

Suggested cooking time: 12 minutes

Time total: 22 minutes

What to Use

- Pepper (as desired)

- Salt (as desired)

- Extra virgin olive oil (2 T)

- Parmesan cheese (2 T)

- Feta cheese (.5 c crumbled)

- Mushrooms (4 sliced)

- Spinach (1 bunch chopped, rinsed)

- Roma tomatoes (2 chopped)

- Whole wheat pita (6, 6 in.)

- Sun-dried tomato pesto (6 oz.)

What to Do

- Ensure your oven is heated to 350°F.

- Top one side of each pita using the sun-dried tomato pesto before placing them face-up on a baking sheet. Top with mushrooms, spinach, and tomatoes before adding the parmesan and feta cheese and topping with olive oil and seasoning as desired.

- Place the baking sheet in the oven and let the pita bake until they are crisp which should take approximately 10 minutes.

- Quarter the pita prior to serving.

Snack: Celery Fries

Makes enough for: 6

Time required for proper preparation: 10 minutes

Suggested cooking time: 25 minutes

Time total: 35 minutes

What to Use

- Black pepper (.25 tsp.)

- Salt (.5 tsp.)

- Olive oil (2 T)

- Root celery (1.5 lbs.)

What to Do

- Start by making sure your oven is heated to 400°F.

- Cut the celery into strips before adding to a mixing bowl, coating in oil, and seasoning with salt and pepper. Shake well.

- Add the fries to a baking sheet and place them in the oven to bake for 20 minutes.

Dinner: Asparagus and Lemon Chicken

Makes enough for: 4

Time required for proper preparation: 5 minutes

Suggested cooking time: 25 minutes

Time total: 30 minutes

What to Use

- Coconut oil (2 T divided)

- Pepper (as desired)

- Salt (as desired)

- Chicken stock (1 c)

- Dijon mustard (1 T)

- Lemon zest (.5 lemon)

- Lemon juice (3 T)

- Garlic (2 cloves crushed)

- Asparagus stalks (1 lb.)

- Tapioca flour (.25 c)

- Chicken breast (4 skinless, boneless)

What to Do

- Start by placing each of the chicken breasts between a pair of pieces of plastic wrap before pounding them down until they are about .25 inches thick each.

- Add the pepper, salt, and flour to a mixing bowl before adding in the chicken and ensuring it is well-coated.

- Add 1 T of the oil to a skillet before placing it on top of a burner turned to a high/medium heat. Once the oil is thoroughly heated, add in the chicken and let it cook approximately 5 minutes per side or until it reaches an internal temperature of at least 165 degrees. Remove it from the skillet while you cook the asparagus.

- Add the rest of the oil to the skillet before adding in the asparagus stalks and letting them cook for 60 seconds before adding in the garlic and letting it cook for yet another minute.

- While it is cooking, mix together the mustard and lemon juice in a small cup and whisk well. Add the results to the skillet and turn the heat up to allow the liquid to boil.

- Once it does so, reduce the heat and allow it to boil for approximately 3 minutes until the asparagus becomes tender.

- Plate the chicken and top with the asparagus and the excess liquid.

Dessert: Coconut Cream Macaroons

Makes enough for: 5

Time required for proper preparation: 15 minutes

Suggested cooking time: 55 minutes

Time total: 70 minutes

What to Use

- Heavy cream (3 oz.)

- Cream cheese (9 oz.)

- Vanilla (1 tsp.)

- Egg whites (4 or 5)

- Cream of tartar (.25 tsp.)

- Erythritol (1 c)

- Salt (.125 tsp.)

- Dried coconut (18 oz.)

- Unsweetened white chocolate syrup (as desired)

- Semi-sweet chocolate chips (as desired)

What to Do

- Preheat oven to 325°F.

- Separate the yolks from the eggs.

- Whisk the egg whites, vanilla, cream of tartar, and the salt together, occasionally sprinkling in the erythritol. Whisk until the mixture peaks.

- Add coconut to the egg white mixture. Mix and set bowl aside.

- In a separate bowl, mix together the chocolate syrup, cream cheese, and the heavy cream. Mix the ingredients well.

- Add the ingredients from the other bowl and mix all ingredients together.

- Add the chocolate chips after everything else is mixed. Scoop mixture onto a cookie sheet. Bake in a preheated oven for about 25 minutes. Turn the oven off and let the cookies remain in the oven for another 30 minutes, so they will dry.

DAY 7

Breakfast: Breakfast Casserole

Makes enough for: 6

Time required for proper preparation: 20 minutes

Suggested cooking time: 6 hours

Time total: 6 hours and 20 minutes

What to Use

- Ground black pepper (as desired)

- Sea salt (as desired)

- Dry mustard (.5 tsp.)

- Paprika (.5 tsp.)

- Pepper (.5 tsp.)

- Garlic powder (1 tsp.)

- Scallions (6 diced)

- Fat-free milk (1 c)

- Egg whites (14)

- Mushrooms (8 oz. diced)

- Bell pepper (1 diced)

- Cheddar cheese (1 c shredded)

- Hash browns (1 packaged frozen)

What to Do

- Ensure the slow cooker has been sprayed down using cooking spray to ensure nothing sticks.

- Layer in the mushrooms, onions, bell peppers, and potatoes plus the cheese so that it makes two or three distinct layers.

- Combine the dry mustard, garlic powder, paprika, pepper, salt, milk, and egg whites together in a mixing bowl and mix well before adding the results to the slow cooker.

- Cover the slow cooker and let it cook on low heat for 6 hours.

Lunch: Cabbage Soup

Makes enough for: 9

Time required for proper preparation: 30 minutes

Suggested cooking time: 3 hours

Time total: 3 hours and 30 minutes

What to Use

- Salt (as needed)
- Pepper (as needed)
- Cabbage (8 c sliced)
- Beef broth (5 c)
- Cauliflower (2 c riced)
- Marinara sauce (16 oz.)
- Oregano (.5 tsp. dried)
- Parsley (1 tsp. dried)
- Stew beef (2 lbs.)
- Shallots (.5 c chopped)
- Onion (.5 c chopped)
- Garlic (2 cloves minced)
- Extra virgin olive oil (2 T)

What to Do

- Add the olive oil to a skillet before placing it on top of a burner set to a high-medium heat before adding in the garlic, shallot, and onion. Let them soften. Add in the beef and let it cook for about 5 minutes, stirring regularly to ensure it browns evenly. Add in the marinara sauce and season as desired before adding in the cauliflower and mixing well.

- Add the result to the slow cooker before adding in the remaining ingredients and mixing well.

- Adjust the slow cooker temperature to high and leave it be, covered, for 3 hours.

Snack: Low Carb Quesadilla

Makes enough for: 3

Time required for proper preparation: 10 minutes

Suggested cooking time: 15 minutes

Time total: 25 minutes

What to Use - Tortillas

- Salt (.5 tsp.)

- Coconut flour (1 T)

- Psyllium husk powder (2 tsp.)

- Cream cheese (6 oz.)

- Eggs (2 large)

- Egg whites (2)

What to Use - Filling

- Olive oil (1 tsp.)

- Leafy greens (1 oz.)

- Cheese (.25 lbs. shredded)

- Low carb tortillas (6)

What to Do - Tortillas

- Start by making sure your oven is heated to 400°F.

- Using a hand mixer, whisk together the eggs whites and the eggs for 3 minutes before adding in the cream cheese and whisking well.

- Using a small bowl, combine in the coconut flour, psyllium husk, and salt. Slowly add the results to the batter, whisking all the while.

- Let the batter thicken until it resembles traditional pancake batter, the exact amount of time will vary based on the type of psyllium husk used.

- Spread the batter onto a lined cooking sheet so that it makes 6.25-inch-thick circles.

- Place the baking sheet onto the upper oven rack and bake for 5 minutes.

What to Do - Quesadillas

- Take three of the tortillas and top them with half of the cheese, the greens, and the remaining cheese. Top with the remaining tortillas.

- Add a small amount of oil to a skillet before placing it on the stove over a burner set to a high/medium heat. Once it has heated, add in one of the quesadillas and cook 1 minute per side.

- Repeat with the remaining quesadillas and serve hot.

Dinner: Carbonara

Makes enough for: 4

Time required for proper preparation: 15 minutes

Suggested cooking time: 25 minutes

Time total: 40 minutes

What to Use

- Black pepper (as desired)

- Sea salt (as desired)

- Coconut oil (1 T)

- Parmesan cheese (3 oz.)

- Egg yolks (4)

- Zucchini (2 lbs.)

- Parsley (chopped fine)

- Keto mayonnaise (4 T)

- Heavy whipping cream (1.25 c)

What to Do

- Add the heavy cream to a saucepan before placing it on the stove over a burner turned to high heat. Reduce the heat and let it simmer until it has reduced about 25 percent.

- Cook the bacon in the coconut oil until it is extra crispy. Remove it from the pan and save the fat.

- Combine the mayonnaise and the heavy cream, season as desired, and let it remain on the stove until it is heated all the way through.

- Using a spiralizer, make noodles from the zucchini. A potato peeler will also work.

- Plate the noodles before topping with sauce, bacon, parsley, parmesan cheese, and egg yolks. Top with bacon grease directly prior to serving.

Dessert: Walnut Orange Chocolate Bites

Makes enough for: 8

Time required for proper preparation: 3 hours

Suggested cooking time: 0 minutes

Time total: 3 hours

What to Use

- Extra virgin coconut oil (.25 c)

- Orange peel or orange extract (.5 T)

- Walnuts (1.75 c chopped)

- Cinnamon (1 tsp.)

- Stevia (10-15 drops)

- Cocoa dark chocolate (pieces)

What to Do

- Melt the chocolate with your choice of method.

- Add cinnamon and coconut oil. Sweeten mixture with stevia.

- Pour in fresh orange peel and chopped walnuts.

- In a muffin tin, spoon in mixture.

- Place into the fridge for 1-3 hours until mixture is solid.

DAY 8

Breakfast: Pumpkin Spice Cake

Makes enough for: 10

Time required for proper preparation: 15 minutes

Suggested cooking time: 2 hours and 30 minutes

Time total: 2 hours and 45 minutes

What to Use

- Vanilla extract (1 tsp.)

- Coconut oil (.25 c melted)

- Cinnamon (1 tsp.)

- Eggs (4)

- Pumpkin puree (1 c)

- Salt (.25 tsp.)

- Cloves (.25 tsp.)

- Baking powder (2 tsp.)

- Whey protein powder (.25 c)

- Coconut flour (.3 c)

- Swerve (.75 c granulated)

- Pecans (1.5 c raw)

- Ginger (1.25 tsp.)

What to Do

- Line the inside of your slow cooker using a parchment paper.

- Add the pecans to your food processor and run them through it until they become a coarse meal. Place the result into a bowl before mixing in salt, cloves, ginger, cinnamon, baking powder, whey protein powder, coconut flour, and swerve and whisk well.

- Mix in the vanilla, oil, eggs, and pumpkin puree and combine thoroughly. Pour the results into your slow cooker.

- Adjust the slow cooker temperature to low and leave it covered for about hours. When finished, the top of the cake should be slightly firm.

Lunch: Thai Fish

Makes enough for: 4

Time required for proper preparation: 10 minutes

Suggested cooking time: 20 minutes

Time total: 30 minutes

What to Use

- Olive oil (2 T)

- Cilantro (.5 c chopped)

- Coconut cream (1 can)

- Red curry paste (2 T)

- Coconut oil (4 T)

- Pepper (as desired)

- Salt (as desired)

- Whitefish (1.5 lbs.)

What to Do

- Start by making sure your oven is heated to 400°F.

- Add the fish to a baking dish before seasoning as needed and topping with 1T coconut oil per fish portion.

- In a small bowl, combine the cilantro, curry paste, and coconut cream before using it to top the fish.

- Place the baking dish in the oven and let it cook for 20 minutes.

Snack: Parmesan Zucchini Tomato Gratin

Makes enough for: 6

Time required for proper preparation: 10 minutes

Suggested cooking time: 40 minutes

Time total: 50 minutes

What to Use

- Basil (2 tsp.)

- Garlic powder (1 tsp.)

- Salt (.5 tsp.)

- Garlic (2 T minced)

- Olive oil (2 T)

- Onion (.5 c chopped)

- Parmesan cheese (.5 c shredded)

- Tomatoes (2)

- Zucchini (3)

What to Do

- Ensure your oven is preheated to 350°F.

- Sauté onions until translucent and fragrant. Add garlic, sautéing for 1 to 2 minutes longer. Pour mixture into the bottom of a casserole dish.

- With a knife, slice tomatoes and zucchinis.

- Layer zucchini and tomatoes, alternating layers.

- Drizzle veggies with olive oil, sprinkle with seasonings and cover with Parmesan cheese.

- Bake for 40 minutes until gratin turns a light brown.

Dinner: Stir Fry with Cabbage

Makes enough for: 4

Time required for proper preparation: 15 minutes

Suggested cooking time: 30 minutes

Time total: 45 minutes

What to Use

- Wasabi paste (.5 T)

- Keto mayonnaise (1 c)

- Sesame oil (1 T)

- Ginger (1 T grated)

- Chili flakes (1 tsp.)

- Scallions (3 sliced)

- Garlic (2 cloves)

- White wine vinegar (1 T)

- Black pepper (.25 tsp. ground)

- Onion powder (1 tsp.)

- Salt (1 tsp.)

- Beef (1.3 lbs. ground)

- Coconut oil (5 oz. grass fed)

- Cabbage (1.6 lbs. shredded)

What to Do

- Add 3 oz. coconut oil to a frying pan before placing the pan on a burner set to a high/medium heat.

- Add the cabbage to the frying pan and let it cook, taking care to prevent it from browning. Season using vinegar and spices before continuing to stir and fry an additional 2 minutes before removing the cabbage from heat.

- Add the remainder of the butter to the frying pan before adding in the ginger, chili flakes, and garlic and sautéing for 3 minutes.

- Add in the meat and let it brown before reducing the heat to medium and adding in the cabbage and scallions. Season using pepper, salt, and sesame oil and ensure everything is hot prior to serving.

- Combine the wasabi paste and the mayo and add the results to the stir fry prior to serving.

Dessert: Oatmeal Chocolate Bites

Makes enough for: 8

Time required for proper preparation: 65 minutes

Suggested cooking time: 0 minutes

Time total: 65 minutes

What to Use

- Flaxseed (.25 c ground)

- Chocolate chips (.5 c)

- Almond butter (.5 c)

- Rolled oats (1 c)

- Raw honey (.3 c)

What to Do

- Mix all the recipe components together.

- Roll out tsp. sized balls onto a tray lined with parchment paper.

- Freeze balls for 1 hour.

- Freeze for up to 1 month.

DAY 9

Breakfast: Blueberry and Beet Greens Smoothie

Makes enough for: 1

Time required for proper preparation: 5 minutes

Suggested cooking time: 0 minutes

Time total: 5 minutes

What to Use

- Stevia (as desired)
- Cinnamon (.5 tsp.)
- Beet greens (2 c chopped, stems removed)
- Banana (.5 medium, frozen, peeled)
- Blueberries (.5 c peeled)
- Green apple (1 cored, halved)
- Water (1 c)

What to Do

- Blend all of the ingredients until they reach the desired consistency (typically for about 45 seconds on a high setting for a blender that is at least 1000 watts). Make sure to add the liquids in before the solids.

Lunch: Fish Tacos

Makes enough for: 4

Time required for proper preparation: 15 minutes

Suggested cooking time: 25 minutes

Time total: 40 minutes

What to Use

- Tomato (1 chopped)
- Avocado (1 diced)
- Cilantro (.25 c chopped)
- Lime juice (.5 limes)
- Chili pepper (1 chopped, seeded)
- Garlic clove (2 chopped)
- Coconut oil (2 T)
- Shrimp (.6 lbs. peeled)
- Cumin (.5 tsp. ground)
- Cheese (.5 lbs. shredded)

What to Do

- Start by making sure your oven is heated to 400°F.

- Combine the cumin with the cheese and add the results in eight piles onto a lined baking sheet.

- The goal is to cook the cheese until it starts to form brown patches which should take about 15 minutes.

- Let the cheese cool briefly before placing each on a rack so that it will form into a general taco shape.

- While they are cooling, place a pan on the stove over a burner turned to medium-high heat and add in the coconut oil before letting it warm up and adding in the shrimp.

- Let the shrimp cook until they have turned a rich pink and season as needed.

- Combine all ingredients, serve, and enjoy.

Snack: Flaxseed Crackers and Keto Spinach and Artichoke Dip

Makes enough for: 6

Time required for proper preparation: 10 minutes

Suggested cooking time: 60 minutes

Time total: 70 minutes

What to Use

- Flax seeds (1 c)

- Red pepper flakes (.5 tsp., optional)

- Water (1 c)

- Onion powder (.5 tsp., optional)

- Rosemary (.5 tsp., optional)

- Garlic powder (.5 tsp., optional)

What to Do

- Dump flaxseeds into a bowl. Put in the fridge for up to eighteen hours.

- Take the flax seeds and place them on a sheet of parchment paper. Roll as thin as you can get them.

- Your oven needs to be set to 275°F and the seeds cooked for an hour on the paper they are sitting on.

Dinner: Chicken Casserole

Makes enough for: 4

Time required for proper preparation: 15 minutes

Suggested cooking time: 30 minutes

Time total: 45 minutes

What to Use

- Coconut oil (2 T)

- Pepper (as desired)

- Salt (as desired)

- Garlic (1 clove chopped)

- Feta cheese (.5 lbs. diced)

- Olives (.5 c pitted)

- Heavy whipping cream (1.5 c)

- Green pesto (4 oz.)

- Chicken breast (1.5 lbs. separated)

What to Do

- Start by making sure your oven is heated to 400°F.

- Season the chicken as desired before adding the coconut oil to a frying pan and placing the pan on the stove over a burner turned to a medium/high heat. Add the chicken once the coconut oil has melted. Let the chicken cook until it turns a golden brown.

- In a mixing bowl, combine the heavy cream and the pesto and mix well.

- Place the chicken, garlic, feta cheese, and olives in a baking dish and top with the pesto mixture.

- Place the baking dish into the oven and let it cook for 30 minutes.

Dessert: Vanilla Granola with Cinnamon

Makes enough for: 12

Time required for proper preparation: 20 minutes

Suggested cooking time: 2 hours

Time total: 2 hours and 20 minutes

What to Use

- Swerve (.5c)

- Salt (1 tsp.)

- Pumpkin seeds (1 c)

- Raw almonds (.5c)

- Raw walnuts (.5c)

- Vanilla extract (1 tsp.)

- Raw pecans (.5c)

- Raw hazelnuts (.5c)

- Raw sunflower seeds (1 c)

- Vanilla Stevia (1 tsp)

- Ground cinnamon (1 tsp)

- Unsweetened shredded coconut (1 c)

- Coconut oil (.3 c)

What to Do

- Set the cooker to sauté then add the coconut oil and melt. When melted, add the vanilla extract and Stevia. Stir well before adding coconut, seeds, and nuts. Stir mixture well to coat all ingredients.

- In a bowl, whisk the salt, cinnamon, and swerve then sprinkle with seeds and nuts.

- Close and seal the lid. Set on slow and cook low for 2 hours. Stir every 30 minutes.

- When done, quick-release the pressure. Spread onto a baking pan to cool and store in an airtight container.

DAY 10

Breakfast: Spinach Frittata

Makes enough for: 4

Time required for proper preparation: 5 minutes

Suggested cooking time: 30 minutes

Time total: 35 minutes

What to Use

- Black pepper (as desired)
- Sea salt (as desired)
- Coconut oil (2 T)
- Eggs (8 large, organic)
- Cheese (5.3 oz. shredded)
- Bacon (5.3 oz.)
- Spinach (8 oz.)
- Whipping cream (1 c)

What to Do

- In a small bowl, whisk together the cream, eggs, and your desired seasonings.

- Heat your oven to 350°F.

- Add the bacon to your skillet and place it on the stove over a burner turned to a high/medium heat. Let it cook until it has almost reached your desired level of crispness before adding in the spinach and letting it cook for between 30 and 45 seconds.

- Add all of the ingredients to a baking dish that has been pre-greased and top with the cheese.

- Place the baking dish in the oven and let it cook for about 30 minutes.

- Let it cook for 5 minutes prior to serving.

Lunch: Lamb Meat Pie

Makes enough for: 6

Time required for proper preparation: 30 minutes

Suggested cooking time: 40 minutes

Time total: 70 minutes

What to Use - Crust

- Sesame seeds (.25 c)

- Almond flour (.75 c)

- Powdered psyllium husk (1 T)

- Coconut flour (.25 c)

- Coconut oil (2 T)

- Baking powder (1 tsp)

- Water (.25 c)

- Large egg (1)

- Salt (.25 tsp)

What to Use - Filling

- Sharp cheddar cheese (6 oz)

- Onion (1 finely chopped)

- Cottage cheese (8 oz)

- Coconut oil (2 T)

- Garlic clove (1 chopped)

- Pepper (as needed)

- Salt (as needed)

- Ground lamb (1.5 lbs.)

- Water (.5 c)

- Basil (1 T)

- Ajvar relish (4 T)

What to Do

- Ensure your oven is on and turned to 350°F.

- Place the coconut oil in a frying pan before setting it on the stove above a burner set to a medium/high heat.

- Add in the onion along with the garlic and let it cook for 3 minutes. Add in the lamb and let it brown before seasoning with oregano, basil, salt, and pepper as needed.

- Add in the water along with the ajvar relish. Turn the heat down to low and simmer for 20 minutes.

- Add all of the crust ingredients to a food processor. Process it until it forms a ball of dough.

- Line a springform with parchment paper and add in the dough before placing it in the oven and baking it for 15 minutes.

- Add the results from the skillet to the dough, top with cottage and shredded cheese and bake for 30 minutes.

- Let it cool for 5 minutes prior to serving.

Snack: Chocolate Muffins

Makes enough for: 12

Time required for proper preparation: 10 minutes

Suggested cooking time: 15 minutes

Time total: 25 minutes

What to Use

- Apple cider vinegar (5 milliliters)
- Coconut oil (25 milliliters)
- Caramel syrup (50 milliliters)
- Cocoa powder (5 oz.)
- Golden flaxseed (25 oz.)
- Cinnamon (1 T)
- Baking powder (.5 tsp.)
- Salt (.5 tsp.)
- Slivered almonds (4.5 oz.)

What to Do

- Preheat oven to 350°F.

- Mix all the dry ingredients (except for the almonds) together in a bowl.

- Mix all wet ingredients together in a bowl.

- Combine the dry and wet ingredients together.

- Pour mixture into muffin liners.

- Sprinkle almond slivers on top of each muffin.

- Bake the muffins for 15 minutes.

Dinner: Mandarin Chicken

Makes enough for: 12

Time required for proper preparation: 20 minutes

Suggested cooking time: 4 hours

Time total: 4 hours and 20 minutes

What to Use

- Salt (as needed)

- Pepper (as needed)

- Sesame oil (1 tsp.)

- Fish sauce (2 T)

- Swerve (1 T)

- Lime juice (1 T)

- Red chili (.5 tsp.)

- Ginger (1 T)

- Garlic (1 tsp. minced)

- Mandarin orange slices (1 c no sugar added)

- Chinese 5 spice powder (1 T)

- Chicken thighs (6)

- Xanthan gum (.5 tsp.)

What to Do

- Mix together the salt and the 5-spice powder in a small bowl before rubbing the results on the chicken.

- Place the chicken in a pan and place the pan on the oven over a burner turned to a high/medium heat and let each side sear for about 3 minutes.

- Place the chicken on the bottom of the slow cooker and then add in the rest of the ingredients, with the exception of the xanthan gum and coating it well. Adjust the slow cooker temperature to high and leave it be, covered, for about 4 hours.

- Remove the chicken from the slow cooker and remove the chicken from the thighs with two forks.

- Take the sauce from the slow cooker and pour it into a blender. Blend well and serve with the chicken.

Dessert: Chocolate Mint Smoothie

Makes enough for: 1

Time required for proper preparation: 5 minutes

Suggested cooking time: 0 minutes

Time total: 5 minutes

What to Use

- Ice cubes (6)

- Your choice of sweetener (as desired)

- Coconut milk (1.75 c)

- Chocolate whey protein (1 scoop)

- Avocado (.5)

- Erythritol (2 T)

- Cocoa powder (1 T)

- Mint leaves (6 fresh, torn)

- MCT oil (1 T)

What to Do

- Slice the avocado lengthwise before removing the seeds and the skin. Add the sliced avocado along with the remaining ingredients to your blender.

- Cream the coconut milk: This is a simple process. All you need to do is place the can of coconut milk in the refrigerator overnight. The next morning, open the can and spoon out the coconut milk that has solidified. Don't shake the can before opening. Discard the liquids.

- Add all of the ingredients, except the ice cubes, to the blender and blend on low speed until pureed. Thin with water as needed.

- Add in the ice cubes and blend until the smoothie reaches your desired consistency.

DAY 11

Breakfast: Anti-inflammatory Turmeric Smoothie

Makes enough for: 1

Time required for proper preparation: 5 minutes

Suggested cooking time: 0 minutes

Time total: 5 minutes

What to Use

- Frozen pineapple (1 c)

- Coconut oil (1 tsp.)

- Peeled, chopped fresh ginger (1 tsp.)

- Cold water (1-1.5 c)

- Frozen mango (1 c)

- Turmeric powder (.25 c)

- Water (.5 c)

- Black pepper (.75 tsp.)

What to Do

- Place all the ingredients in a blender and blend until super smooth. Enjoy!

- Mix the turmeric and water in a pan over low heat, stirring until a paste is formed.

- Once you have a paste, stir in the black pepper.

- Cool and store in a glass jar in the fridge for up to 2 weeks.

Lunch: Brussels Sprouts Surprise

Makes enough for: 12

Time required for proper preparation: 15 minutes

Suggested cooking time: 30 minutes

Time total: 45 minutes

What to Use

- Coconut oil (2 T melted)

- Almond flour (1 c)

- Parmesan cheese (4 oz. grated)

- Heavy cream (2 c)

- Garlic (2 T minced)

- Thyme (2 tsp.)

- Cheddar cheese (8 oz.)

- Brussels sprouts (2 lb. sliced thin)

What to Do

- Ensure your oven is heated to 350°F.

- If you don't want to slice the Brussels sprouts by hand, a food processor will also do the trick.

- In a mixing bowl, combine the Brussels sprouts with the garlic, thyme, and cheese and mix well.

- Add the results to a prepared casserole dish and spread evenly.

- In a separate bowl, combine the coconut oil, parmesan cheese, and almond flour and mix until it begins to crumble.

- Add this mixture to the top of the casserole dish and spread evenly.

- Add the dish to the oven for 30 minutes or until the crust has browned and the cheese is bubbling.

Snack: Stuffed Avocado

Makes enough for: 2

Time required for proper preparation: 5 minutes

Suggested cooking time: 0 minutes

Time total: 5 minutes

What to Use

- Salt (as desired)

- Pepper (as desired)

- Coconut oil (2 T)

- Lemon juice (2 T)

- Cayenne pepper (.25 tsp.)

- Garlic powder (.5 tsp.)

- Onion powder (.5 tsp.)

- Paprika (1 tsp.)

- Thyme (1 tsp. dried)

- Sour cream (2 T)

- Mayonnaise (.25 c)

- Chicken (1.5 c cooked)

- Avocados (2 medium sliced)

What to Do

- Shred the chicken into a small mixing bowl before mixing in the cayenne pepper, garlic powder, coconut oil, onion powder, paprika, thyme, sour cream, and mayonnaise. Mix well. Season with lemon juice, salt, and pepper as desired.

- Scoop out the middle of each avocado, leaving approximately .5 inches of space around the outside.

- Add the removed avocado to the mixing bowl and mix well.

- Add the results back into the scoop out avocados prior to serving.

Dinner: Chicken and Veggies

Makes enough for: 4

Time required for proper preparation: 10 minutes

Suggested cooking time: 25 minutes

Time total: 35 minutes

What to Use

- Coconut milk (14 oz.)

- Ground coriander (.25 tsp.)

- Ground cumin (1 pinch)

- Green curry paste (2 T)

- Grated ginger (1 piece)

- Chopped chilies (3)

- Olive oil (2 T)

- Minced garlic cloves (3)

- Chopped basil (.5 c)

- Chopped cilantro (.5 c)

- Chopped spinach (4 c)

- Coconut aminos (1 T)

- Pepper

- Salt

- Chicken pieces (8)

- Cubed eggplant (1)

- Cubed squash (6 c)

What to Do

- Turn the Instant Pot on and add the oil, coriander, cumin, chilies, ginger, and garlic. Cook for a minute.

- Add the coconut milk and curry paste and cook for 4 minutes before adding the pepper, salt, eggplant, squash, and chicken.

- Cover the pot and cook the meal on a high setting for 20 minutes.

- Take the lid off at this time and add the cilantro, basil, aminos, and spinach. Divide this up and serve.

Dessert: Vanilla Pound Cake

Makes enough for: 12

Time required for proper preparation: 15 minutes

Suggested cooking time: 60 minutes

Time total: 75 minutes

What to Use

- Whole wheat flour (1.75 c)

- Salt (.25 tsp.)

- Baking powder (.75 tsp.)

- Sugar (1.3 c)

- Coconut oil (3.5 T)

- Light cream cheese (8 oz.)

- Almond extract (1 tsp.)

- Vanilla extract (2.5 tsp.)

- Egg whites (3)

- Eggs (2)

What to Do

- Start by making sure your oven is heated to 350°F.

- Prepare a loaf pan (9-inch) by spraying it with cooking spray.

- Whisk together the almond extract, vanilla extract, egg whites, and eggs in a small mixing bowl and set to one side.

- In a larger mixing bowl, beat together the coconut oil and cream cheese with the help of an electric mixer. Beat in the salt, baking powder, and sugar until blended as well.

- Add in the egg mixture and flour slowly, starting and finishing with the flour. Beat well.

- Add the batter to the loaf pan and bake for 60 minutes. You will know it is finished when you can stick a toothpick into the center and have it come out clean.

- Allow the cake to cool on a wire rack prior to serving.

DAY 12

Breakfast: Scrambled Eggs with Avocado and Bacon

Makes enough for: 4

Time required for proper preparation: 5 minutes

Suggested cooking time: 10 minutes

Time total: 15 minutes

What to Use

- Pepper (as desired)
- Salt (as desired)
- Bacon (2 oz.)
- Olive oil (1 tsp.)
- Avocado (.5 peeled)
- Eggs (2)

What to Do

- Preheat the oven to 350°F.
- In a small pot, place the eggs and add cold water until the eggs are completely covered by roughly 1 inch of water. Add

the pot to the stove above a boiler turned to a high/medium heat and let the water boil.

- After the water has boiled, remove the pot from the stove and let it cool for roughly 10 minutes and then drain the pot.

- Fill a large bowl with cold water and dunk the eggs briefly into it to make them easier to peel.

- Peel and prepare the eggs as preferred before placing them in a bowl. They should be warm, not hot.

- Split the eggs and remove the yolks and discard them.

- In a mixing bowl, combine the eggs, oil, and avocado and mix well before seasoning with pepper and salt as needed.

- Place the bacon on a baking sheet and place the baking sheet in the oven for 5 minutes.

- Once the bacon is no longer hot to the touch, break each piece in half and portion out a half per serving of eggs.

Lunch: Prosciutto and Beets with Onion Dressing

Makes enough for: 6

Time required for proper preparation: 25 minutes

Suggested cooking time: 45 minutes

Time total: 70 minutes

What to Use

- Black pepper (.5 tsp.)
- Salt (.5 tsp.)
- Extra virgin olive oil (1 T + 1 tsp.)
- Salad greens (14 c)
- Chives (1 T chopped)
- Mayonnaise 92 T)
- White wine vinegar (2 T)
- Buttermilk (.25 c)
- Dried thyme (.25 tsp.)
- Onion (1 sliced)
- Beets (12 oz.)
- Prosciutto (2 oz. cut into squares)

What to Do

- Ensure your oven is heated to 400°F.

- Prepare a baking sheet by covering it with .5 tsp. olive oil.

- Place the prosciutto squares onto the baking sheet and bake them for 5 minutes.

- Place them on a wire rack to cool.

- Place the beets into a saucepan and cover them with 2 inches of water. Place the pan on a burner set to high heat and let it boil before turning the heat to low and letting them cook for 20 minutes.

- Drain the beets, let them cool, remove the skin, and cut them into wedges.

- Add the oil to a saucepan before placing the pan on the stove over a burner set to a low/medium heat. Add in the pepper, salt, and thyme before covering the pan and cooking for 10 minutes, stirring regularly.

- Uncover the pan and let it cook for an additional 8 minutes before removing the pan from heat and letting it sit for 10 minutes.

- Separate out a fourth of the onion and add the rest to a food processor before adding in the chives, mayonnaise, vinegar, and buttermilk and processing thoroughly.

- Combine all ingredients prior to serving.

Snack: Spinach and Kale Smoothie with Jelly and Peanut Butter

Makes enough for: 2

Time required for proper preparation: 5 minutes

Suggested cooking time: 0 minutes

Time total: 5 minutes

What to Use

- Organic milk (.5 c)

- Plain Greek yogurt (.5 c)

- Kale (.5 c)

- Baby spinach (.5 c)

- Banana (1 peeled)

- Strawberries (.5 c)

- Peanut butter (1 T)

What to Do

- Add all of the ingredients to your blender and blend well.

- Serve chilled and enjoy.

Dinner: Ratatouille Kebabs

Makes enough for: 4

Time required for proper preparation: 35 minutes

Suggested cooking time: 10 minutes

Time total: 45 minutes

What to Use

- Tomato paste (2 T)

- Red onion (1 chopped)

- Yellow bell pepper (1 chopped)

- Zucchini (1 sliced)

- Eggplant (6 oz. sliced)

- Cherry tomatoes (16)

- Ground pepper (.5 tsp.)

- Oregano (1 T chopped)

- Lemon juice (2 T)

- Lemon zest (1 tsp.)

- Extra virgin olive oil (4 T divided)

- Tofu (14 oz. drained)

What to Do

- Ensure the tofu is dry before cutting it into cubes.

- Add the pepper, oregano, lemon juice, lemon zest, and 1 T extra virgin olive oil together in a large bowl before adding in the tofu and letting it soak for at least 24 hours.

- Turn your grill to medium heat.

- In a large bowl, combine the pepper, the remaining extra virgin olive oil, onion, bell pepper, zucchini, eggplant, and tomatoes together.

- Add all of the ingredients onto skewers.

- Mix the tomato paste into the used marinade and coat the skewers with it prior to cooking.

- Add the skewers to the grill and let each side cook for roughly 4 minutes until it begins to blacken.

Dessert: Carrot Cake Muffins

Makes enough for: 12

Time required for proper preparation: 10 minutes

Suggested cooking time: 25 minutes

Time total: 35 minutes

What to Use

- Whole wheat flour (1.25 c + .5 c)
- Salt (.25 tsp)
- Cinnamon (1 tsp)
- Baking soda (.25 tsp)
- Baking powder (1 tsp)
- Sour cream (.25 c)
- Cream cheese (.5 c)
- Coconut oil (2 T)
- Sugar (2.5 T)
- Vanilla (1 tsp)
- Brown sugar (2.5 T)
- Egg (1)
- Carrots (1 c)

- Pineapple (.5 c crushed)

What to Do

- Set your oven ahead of time to 375°F.

- Place muffin cup into a 12-slot muffin tin.

- In a small mixing bowl, combine the sugar, cream cheese, and egg together and mix well before adding in the pineapple as well as the carrots.

- In a separate bowl, mix together the sour cream, coconut oil, sugar, and brown sugar and blend well before mixing in the vanilla.

- Ensure there is space in the dry ingredients for the wet ingredients before combining the two bowls and mixing well. Take care not to overmix.

- Fill the muffin tins with the results, taking care to leave a room in each space for the baked muffin to rise.

- Add the tin to the preheated oven and bake for 20 minutes. The muffins will be fully cooked when you can stick a toothpick into the center of the center muffins and it comes out clean.

- Allow the muffins 20 minutes to cool before serving.

DAY 13

Breakfast: Breakfast Burritos

Makes enough for: 2

Time required for proper preparation: 15 minutes

Suggested cooking time: 15 minutes

Time total: 30 minutes

What to Use

- Eggs (2)
- Water (.5 c)
- Flax seeds (4 tsp. gr
- Salt (1 pinch)
- Egg whites (2)
- Coconut oil (1 tsp.)
- Spinach leaves (1 handful)
- Tilapia (.25 c baked)
- Onion (.25 c diced)
- Red bell pepper (.25 c diced)
- Avocado (1 diced)

What to Do

- Preheat the broiler on your oven.

- Heat a skillet using medium heat and coat it with cooking spray.

- Mix together the eggs, egg whites, salt, flax seeds, and water.

- Pour 50 percent of the mixture into the pan and let it cook for 2 minutes.

- Set the skillet below the broiler and leave it for 3 minutes. You will know it is time when the tortilla begins to bubble.

- Take the tortilla out of the pan and place it on some aluminum foil before repeating the process with the remaining tortilla mixture.

- Ensure your oven is preheated to 400°F.

- Place a pan on medium heat and put the coconut oil inside of it. Mix in the peppers and onions and let them sauté for 5 minutes until they have started to soften.

- Mix in the spinach and let it wilt.

- Mix all of the ingredients together and bake for 5 minutes to let them set.

- Serve hot and enjoy.

Lunch: Asian Lettuce Wraps

Makes enough for: 4

Time required for proper preparation: 5 minutes

Suggested cooking time: 10 minutes

Time total: 15 minutes

What to Use

- Lime (1 wedged)
- Cilantro (1 bunch dried)
- Mint (1 bunch (dried)
- Cucumber (1 peeled, sliced thin)
- Lettuce (12 leaves)
- Sesame oil (1 tsp.)
- Soy sauce (3 T)
- Sugar (1 tsp.)
- Red pepper flakes (.5 tsp.)
- Garlic (2 cloves chopped)
- Ginger (2 T chopped)
- Scallions (3 sliced)
- Red pepper (1 seeded, sliced)

- Ground turkey (1 lb.)

- Vegetable oil (1 T)

What to Do

- Add the oil to a skillet before placing the skillet on the stove over a burner turned to a high/medium heat. Crumble the turkey and add it to the skillet to cook for 5 minutes.

- Add in the sugar, red pepper flakes, garlic, ginger, scallion, and red pepper. Turn the heat off and mix in the sesame oil and soy sauce.

- Combine the ingredients as desired prior to serving.

Snack: Green Beans with Roasted Pecans

Makes enough for: 3

Time required for proper preparation: 15 minutes

Suggested cooking time: 20 minutes

Time total: 35 minutes

What to Use

- Red pepper flakes (.5 tsp.)

- Garlic (1 tsp. minced)

- Lemon zest (.5 lemons)

- Parmesan cheese (2 T)

- Pecans (.25 c chopped)

- Olive oil (2 T)

- Green beans (.5 lbs.)

What to Do

- Start by making sure your oven is heated to 400°F.

- Add the pecans to your food processor and process vigorously. Don't worry if they are not all the same size.

- Add the red pepper flakes, minced garlic, lemon zest, parmesan cheese, olive oil, pecans, and green beans together in a mixing bowl and mix well.

- Add the results to a baking sheet that has been covered in tinfoil.

- Place the baking sheet in the oven and let the green beans and pecans bake for about 20 minutes.

- Let the contents of the baking sheet cool for 5 minutes prior to serving.

Dinner: Avocado and Chili Bake

Makes enough for: 4

Time required for proper preparation: 25 minutes

Suggested cooking time: 40 minutes

Time total: 65 minutes

What to Use - Crust

- Water (.25 c)

- Egg (1 large)

- Coconut oil (3 T)

- Salt (1 pinch)

- Baking powder (1 tsp.)

- Psyllium husk (1 T powdered)

- Coconut flour (.25 c)

- Sesame seeds (.25 c)

- Almond flour (.75 c)

What to Use - Filling

- Cheese (1.25 c shredded)

- Cream cheese (.5 c)

- Salt (.25 tsp.)

- Onion powder (.5 tsp.)

- Chili pepper (1 chopped, seeded)

- Cilantro (2 T chopped)

- Eggs (3 large)

- Mayonnaise (1 c)

- Avocado (2 peeled, pitted)

What to Do

- Start by making sure your oven is heated to 350°F.

- Combine the ingredients for the dough together using a food processor and process vigorously until they form a ball of dough.

- Line a 12-inch springform and place the dough into it before placing the dough into the oven and letting it bake for 15 minutes.

- Combine the remaining ingredients in a mixing bowl and mix well before filling the crust.

- Place the springform back into the oven and let it cook for 35 minutes.

Dessert: Banana Gelato

Makes enough for: 2

Time required for proper preparation: 15 minutes

Suggested cooking time: 15 minutes

Time total: 30 minutes

What to Use

- Whipping cream (.25 c)

- Salt (.25 tsp.)

- Vanilla extract (2 tsp.)

- Sugar (.75 c)

- Egg Yolks (5)

- Brown sugar (.25 c)

- Bananas (3 quartered, peeled)

- Skim milk (1.75 c)

What to Do

- In a large saucepan, combine the brown sugar, bananas, and milk and place the pan on a burner turned to medium heat. Add a lid to the pan, turn the heat down, and let it cook for 10 minutes.

- Let everything cool before adding it to a blender and blending well.

- Add the results back to the pan.

- In a large bowl, combine the yolks and sugar.

- Add half of the pan to the bowl and mix well.

- Add everything back into the pan and let it cook for 2 minutes on low heat, stirring well. Mix in the cream, salt, and vanilla.

- Add everything to a container and refrigerate for 48 hours before freezing.

DAY 14

Breakfast: Spinach Roulade with Mushrooms

Makes enough for: 8

Time required for proper preparation: 20 minutes

Suggested cooking time: 20 minutes

Time total: 40 minutes

What to Use

- Eggs (6)

- White Mushrooms (8 Oz. Trimmed and Coarsely Chopped)

- Shiitake Mushrooms (8 Oz.)

- Coconut oil (1 T)

- Spinach (10 Oz. Chopped)

- Cheddar Cheese (1.5 cs Shredded)

- Fresh Parmesan Cheese (.5 c Grated)

- Milk (.67 c)

- Green Onions (2 Sliced Thin)

- Salt (.5 tsp)

- Ground Black Pepper (.25 c)

What to Do

- Heat stove to 350°F.

- Line a jelly-roll pan with a foil.

- Grease the foil.

- Dissolve coconut oil in the skillet on moderate heat.

- Include green onions.

- Cook the onions until wilted or for approximately one minute.

- Blend both types of mushrooms, salt, and pepper in skillet.

- Cook the mushrooms until tender and all liquid had evaporated.

- Take skillet off the heat.

- Puree spinach, eggs, milk, and Parmesan in a blender until smooth.

- Place puree in a jelly-roll pan.

- Smooth out.

- Heat for 8 to 10 minutes or until mixture sets.

- Lift the foil and spread the mushroom mixture on.

- Cover with cheddar, and then add more mushroom mixture over top.

- Using the foil as a guide, roll from one long end.

- Place with the seam side down.

- Heat in the oven until the cheddar melts.

- Slice and serve.

Lunch: Tempeh Triangles with Tahini Carrot Slaw

Makes enough for: 4

Time required for proper preparation: 20 minutes

Suggested cooking time: 5 minutes

Time total: 25 minutes

What to Use

- Pepper (as desired)
- Salt (as desired)
- Cayenne pepper (1 pinch)
- Parsley (.5 c chopped)
- Maple syrup (3 T divided)
- Lemon juice (1 lemon)
- Tahini (2 T)
- Turmeric (.25 tsp powdered)
- Curry powder (1 T)
- Onion (1 diced)
- Carrots (4 c shredded)
- Walnuts (1 T)

- Soy sauce (2 tsp.)

- Olive oil (1 tsp.)

- Liquid smoke (.25 tsp.)

- Tempeh (8 oz. cut into triangles)

What to Do

- Coat a pan in olive oil and place it on the stove above a burner that has been turned to high heat.

- Add the liquid smoke, maple syrup, tamari, and tempeh triangles to the skillet and let it cook for 5 minutes, flipping the tempeh so it absorbs as much liquid as it can.

- After the tempeh has begun to blacken around the edges, remove the skillet from heat before adding in the pepper and walnut pieces.

- In a mixing bowl, combine the onion, raisins, maple syrup, parsley, spices, lemon juice, tahini, and carrots together. Mix well.

- Salads can be made creamier with the addition of more tahini and can be made thinner by adding more apple cider vinegar or lemon juice.

- Add the salad to the salad bowl before adding the tempeh on top. Can be served fresh or chilled.

Snack: Lemon Scones

Makes enough for: 12

Time required for proper preparation: 30 minutes

Suggested cooking time: 15 minutes

Time total: 45 minutes

What to Use

- Lemon juice (1 tsp.)

- Powdered sugar (1 c)

- Buttermilk (.75 c)

- Lemon zest (1 lemon)

- Coconut oil (.25 c)

- Salt (.5 tsp.)

- Baking soda (.5 tsp.)

- Sugar (2 T)

- Flour (2 c +.25 c)

What to Do

- Ensure the oven is heated to 400°F.

- Combine the salt, baking soda, sugar, and 2 c flour together in a mixing bowl.

- Add the results to a food processor, process, add in the coconut oil, and process until crumbles form.

- Mix in the buttermilk and lemon zest.

- Flour a surface and place the dough on top of it.

- Prepare the dough to be baked; the dough should create 12 scones.

- Add the scones to a baking sheet. Add the baking sheet to the oven and cook for approximately 15 minutes.

- Mix the lemon juice and powdered sugar together, add to scones, serve warm and enjoy.

Dinner: Fish Head Soup

Makes enough for: 4

Time required for proper preparation: 45 minutes

Suggested cooking time: 2 hours

Time total: 2 hours and 45 minutes

What to Use

- Black pepper (as desired)

- Salt (as desired)

- Chives (as desired)

- Chilies (as desired)

- Zucchini (3 spiraled to form noodles)

- Coconut aminos (.25 c)

- Ginger (3 T divided)

- Wakame (1 c)

- Green garlic (1 bulb minced)

- Onion (1 small sliced)

- Salmon head (2)

- Salmon tail (2)

What to Do

- Add the fish to the slow cooker along with 2 T of the ginger. Fill the slow cooker with hot water before covering it and letting it cook on high heat for 2 hours.

- Ensure the resulting br oth is strained before adding the broth and the meat to a stock pot.

- Mix in the coconut aminos, wakame, remaining ginger, onions, and garlic before placing the pot on the stove over a burner turned to low heat.

- Let the soup cook for 20 minutes before adding in the zucchini and let it cook for an additional 10 minutes.

- Serve hot, top with chilies and chives, and enjoy.

Dessert: Vanilla Berry Tarts

Makes enough for: 5

Time required for proper preparation: 30 minutes

Suggested cooking time: 30 minutes

Time total: 60 minutes

What to Use - Crust

- Salt (1 pinch)

- Vanilla extract (1 tsp.)

- Cocoa powder (2 T unsweetened)

- Maple syrup (4 T)

- Coconut oil (4 T)

- Baking soda (.5 tsp.)

- Tapioca flour (.25 c + 1 T)

- Coconut flour (.25 c + 1 T)

- Almond flour (1.5 c)

What to Use - Vanilla Cream

- Coconut oil (1 T)

- Vanilla bean (1)

- Vanilla extract (1 tsp.)

- Salt (pinch)

- Tapioca flour (.25 c)

- Maple sugar (.75 c)

- Egg yolks (5)

- Coconut milk (14 oz.)

What to Use - Glaze

- Lime zest (.5 lime)

- Raw honey (1 T)

- Water (1 T)

- Lime juice (2 limes)

What to Use - Toppings

- Strawberries (.3 c)

- Raspberries (.3 c)

- Blackberries (.3 c)

- Blueberries (.3 c)

What to Do

- To make the crust, start by preheating your oven to 325°F.

- Grease 5 tart pans (4 inches).

- Combine all of the crust ingredients in a food processor and process well until it forms a dough.

- Split the dough into fifths and add it to each of the pans, forming it to create a slight bowl shape and poke a few holes in each to prevent it from rising.

- Place the pans in the oven and bake them for 15 minutes. Let them cool for 30 minutes before using.

- To make the vanilla cream, start by adding the coconut milk to a saucepan before placing the pan on the stove on top of a burner set to medium heat. Let it heat until the milk begins to foam, but not boil.

- At the same time, in a mixing bowl, add the maple sugar and egg yolks in a bowl and beat until the results are pale and thick. At this point, reduce the seed of the mixer before adding in the salt as well as the tapioca flour and combining well.

- After the milk has foamed, add half of it to the mixing bowl, mixing on a low speed at the same time. Be careful not to scramble the eggs.

- Add the results to the saucepan and whisk until everything thickens which should be approximately 10 minutes.

- Remove from the stove before adding in the vanilla bean, vanilla extract, and coconut oil and mixing thoroughly.

- Add ice to a large bowl until it is full before placing a glass bowl inside of it. Add the cream from the milk to a sieve into the bowl and cover it to cool for 15 minutes.

- For the glaze, combine all of the glaze ingredients and once the cream and crust have finished cooling, add in the cream and then the berries.

- Top with the glaze and garnish using powdered sugar and mint leaves prior to serving.

Conclusion

Thanks for making it through to the end of *Anti-Inflammatory Diet: The Complete Beginners Guide To Heal The Immune System, Feel Better, and Restore Optimal Health (With Delicious Meal Plan To Get You Started)*. Let's hope it was informative and able to provide you with all of the tools you need to achieve your goals, whatever it is that they may be. Just because you've finished this book doesn't mean there is nothing left to learn on the topic. Expanding your horizons is the only way to find the mastery you seek.

Now that you have made it to the end of this book, you hopefully have an understanding of how to get started with the anti-inflammatory diet, as well as a recipe or two, or three, that you are anxious to try for the first time. Before you go ahead and start giving it your all, however, it is important that you have realistic expectations as to the level of success you should expect in the near future.

Finally, if you found this book useful in any way, a review on Amazon is always appreciated!

Description

Anti-Inflammatory Diet: The Complete Beginners Guide to Heal The Immune System, Feel Better, and Restore Optimal Health

(With Delicious Meal Plan to Get You Started)

Receiving a chronic inflammation diagnosis may seem like the end of the world but you can work through it, and picking up this book and others like it is the first step to drastically improve your quality of life going forward.

This books specifically targets Anti-inflammatory Diet and Meal Plans to help you in getting the best out of your health along with delectable meals. Enjoy carefully crafted meals to optimize your health. See for yourself with a peek at what is ahead for you with these exceptional recipes:

- Carrot Cake Muffins

- Brussels Sprouts Surprise

- Mandarin Chicken

- Avocado Chili Bake

- Banana Gelato

- Fish Tacos

- Breakfast Casserole

- Coconut Cream Macaroons

- Lamb Burger

These delicious treats are only a few of the many recipes you will experience in this lovely Anti-Inflammatory Diet. Make this book one of your most used ones in your digital library today.

THE ANTI-INFLAMMATORY COMPLETE COOKBOOK:

Over 100 Delicious Recipes to Reduce Inflammation, Be Healthy and Feel Amazing

FELICIA RENOLDS

purview. Regardless, there are zero scenarios where the original author or the Publisher can be deemed liable in any fashion for any damages or hardships that may result from any of the information discussed herein.

Additionally, the information in the following pages is intended only for informational purposes and should thus be thought of as universal. As befitting its nature, it is presented without assurance regarding its prolonged validity or interim quality. Trademarks that are mentioned are done without written consent and can in no way be considered an endorsement from the trademark holder.

Introduction

Congratulations on downloading *The Anti-inflammatory Complete Cookbook: Over 100 Delicious Recopies To Reduce Inflammation, Be Healthy and Feel Amazing* and thank you for doing so. Making the decision to change your diet for the better is a big step and one you should be applauded for making. It is also the easiest step, however, as making a true lifestyle change requires commitment and dedication to ensure your new actions stick around long enough to become habits.

Having plenty of choices when it comes to healthy recipes choices is a big part of forming those new habits successfully which is why the following chapters will provide you with plenty of choices regardless of what type of delicious and nutritious recipe you are looking for. Remember, before starting any new diet it is important to check with a dietitian or your primary healthcare provider to ensure you don"t accidentally end up doing more harm than good.

With so many choices out there when it comes to consuming this type of content, it is appreciated that you"ve chosen this one. Plenty of care and effort went into ensuring it contains as many interesting and useful tidbits as possible, please enjoy!

CHAPTER 1

Anti-Inflammatory Diet Rundown

As the name implies, the anti-inflammation diet is a loose collection of rules related to dietary choices designed to reduce the amount of negative chronic inflammation that is known to lead to everything from arthritis, to cancer, to even death. Inflammation is not all bad; however, as when it occurs naturally in the body, it can help the body defend against possible infection as well as heal cuts and wounds.

If it continues for a prolonged period of time, however, it can lead to a host of illnesses and other negative effects (described in detail in chapter 2), some of which can cause serious long term consequences when left unchecked. Luckily, there are numerous easy ways to reduce your levels of overall inflammation including changing your eating habits which is where the anti-inflammatory diet comes into play.

As a part of the inflammation process, the body creates an increased amount of immune cells, white blood cells and a substance known as cytokine as a way to combat infection. There are two primary types of inflammation, the first is a short term variety that presents itself as swelling, heat, some pain, and redness. This is the early phase of inflammation and the symptoms that it brings along with it are caused by the fact that additional blood is flowing to the affected areas in an effort to treat the area as quickly as possible. This ensures that the troubled spot is protected from additional injury as the body works to fend off irritants, damaged cells, pathogens, viruses, and bacteria. Without the inflammation process, even minor cuts and wounds would never heal properly.

Alternately, chronic inflammation happens slowly over a period of months or years while outwardly presenting no noticeable signs of the ever-growing internal issue. This, in turn, creates a gradual shift in the types of cells that exist around the spot of the inflammation as the spot will be constantly in a process of destruction and rebirth, sapping bodily resources and slowly festering and becoming something much worse than whatever the initial injury may have been. This prolonged inflammation can be caused by numerous issues including things like a failure to remove whatever caused the initial inflammation, a misfiring autoimmune response is attacking otherwise healthy cells or the continued presence of a low-level irritant. This will continue until eventually, things get so bad in the inflamed area that the loss of function of a related vital process begins to occur.

What to Do About It

Unfortunately, the average diet of most of the Western world does little to combat chronic inflammation while at the same time doing plenty to help it along. This includes things like a distinct lack of omega-3 fatty acids as they are rarely found in the processed food that is growing increasingly more prevalent worldwide.

Unfortunately, these processed foods do contain a large amount of omega-6 fatty acids and this imbalance specifically is known to cause an increase in the amount of inflammation that a person experiences. What"s worse, the lengths that most people have to go to on a regular basis to ensure they are eating nutritious foods that have not been processed makes it difficult for them to do so regularly.

This is where the anti-inflammatory diet comes in as it makes it easier for individuals to know that what they are eating is actively reducing the inflammatory buildup that they have been experiencing for years prior to the switch. A big reason for this is phytochemicals, naturally occurring chemicals that are found in many of the foods suggested in chapter 3 which are all known to reduce inflammation to various degrees.

Increasing the amount of omega-3 fatty acids that they consume on a regular basis is known to have an even greater benefit for those with rheumatoid arthritis, as consuming more than 3 grams each day has been directly shown to decrease the amount of stiffness, swollenness, and tenderness seen in affected joints. It is also known to have a notable impact on osteoarthritis pain for the same reasons.

A healthy example of a 24-hour anti-inflammation meal plan can be something as simple as steel-cut oatmeal topped with berries or yogurt as well as c of green tea or even coffee. For lunch, a tuna salad sandwich on whole grain bread along with a seasonal fruit smoothie. An afternoon snack could consist of something like walnuts and a bit of dark chocolate; and dinner could be whole grain pasta with an organic tomato sauce and turkey meatballs along with a salad made with walnuts, oranges, and spinach. The day could then be topped with a cranberry and apple pie that avoids the use of the coconut oil.

While the primary use for the diet isn"t weight loss, the focus on natural, healthy meals with reasonable portion sizes means that many individuals do experience a degree of weight loss. This is especially true when it comes to those who previously consumed a higher than average amount of processed foods. This is a naturally occurring phenomenon that comes about when a person decides to eat fewer carbohydrates, unhealthy oils, and trans fats while at the same time filling up on healthy alternatives instead and there is no secret behind it; just clean, healthy eating.

With that being said, it is important to not expect too much too soon as the anti- inflammatory diet is always going to take longer to work than medicines designed directly to affect the problem in question. Rather, the anti-inflammatory diet is a positive lifestyle change that anyone can make that will, over time, make the need for such medicines completely unnecessary. The anti-inflammation diet won"t change your level of inflammation overnight, but it will change it for good.

What to Eat and What to Avoid

When it comes to eating with an eye towards anti-inflammatory foods, there are plenty of options when it comes to avoiding the multitude of harmful products that contain inflammatory producing agents that can broadly be broken down into a handful of categories. Commit the following guidelines for the foods to eat and the foods to avoid to memory and you will be inflammation free in no time flat.

Eat more fiber: Studies show that a diet which is high in fiber is naturally going to create an overall lower level of inflammation because of all of the phytonutrients that natural unprocessed foods including fruits and vegetables have in spades. To ensure you consume 25 grams of fiber per day, make a point of eating lots of blueberries (3.5 grams) bananas (3 grams) onions, eggplant, okra, oatmeal, and barley.

Aim for 9 servings of vegetables and fruits every day: Make a point of consuming a ratio of 2 to 1 vegetables when compared to fruits as too many fruits in a single day can cause your total sugar intake to increase rapidly. A serving is generally considered half a c of cooked vegetables or 1 c of raw vegetables. Both ginger and turmeric are known to fight inflammation as well and both make great seasonings.

Aim for 4 servings of crucifers and alliums each week: Alliums are things like leeks, onions, scallions, and garlic while crucifers comprise numerous vegetables including Brussels sprouts, mustard greens, cauliflower, cabbage, and broccoli. These all contain extremely high levels of antioxidants, which is why only a few each week is enough to significantly lower your risk of inflammation- related cancer when consumed regularly. Remember, 4 servings a week is the minimum when it comes to alliums and crucifers, the more the merrier.

Keep saturated fat to a minimum: In order to start actively reducing the amount of inflammation in your body, it is important that you

216

start keeping a close eye on the number of saturated fats that you are consuming on a daily basis. This means cutting it to 10 percent of the total number of calories that you consume in a day. This means you will likely want to cut down on the red meat and stick with health marinates made from anti-inflammatory spices instead of Coconut oil.

Eat lots of omega-3 fatty acids: As previously discussed, eating more omega-3 fatty acids should be at the top of the list of anyone who is interested in decreasing their inflammation level. In addition to being found in fish, it is also found in large doses in walnuts, flaxseeds and soy, kidney and navy beans. A regular omega-3 supplement is also recommended. When it comes to fish, anchovies, sardines, trout, mackerel, herring, oysters and salmon all contain the highest amounts of omega-3 and you should aim to eat 3 of them each week.

Seek out healthy fats: Fats have gotten somewhat of a bad rap over the years because at some point mainstream society decided to start lumping all fats together. In truth, there are healthy fats which are a good source of energy for those who eschew carbohydrates in favor of a more natural energy solution. This means that plenty of healthy fats like those found in coconut oil, coconut oil and pressed canola oil are a great way to eat healthy while still expelling inflammatory elements from your system.

Avoid product made with corn syrup and/or refined sugar: Studies show that simply adding a daily dose of processed foods to your diet by eating things that are dosed with high amounts of sugar or corn syrup is enough to increase your inflammation levels significantly. Unfortunately, processed food companies understand that the more sugar something has in it the more likely it is to sell which means that it is virtually impossible to find anything processed that has enough sugar or corn syrup in it to cause inflammation in at least 2 full- grown adults. This intense fructose overload is enough to cause inflammation in the lining of blood vessels and should be avoided whenever possible.

Avoid trans-fat: In addition to saturated fats, it is important to avoid trans-fats as often as possible. This means looking at product labels as trans-fats are often hiding under the label of partially hydrogenated oils. Trans-fats are known to cause inflammation in the cell lining of the arteries as well as lower beneficial cholesterol levels which increase that of the harmful variety.

Avoid the wrong types of oil: In general, the healthy fat-based oils that are listed above are a healthy option, all others should be avoided regardless of the health claims they may tout. These oils are often extracted using chemicals that are known to increase inflammation and are rarely disclosed on product labels as they are used in the creation of the product and not added in after the fact. What"s more, they are also typically high in omega-6 fatty acids, decreasing the balance in the body between that and omega-3 fatty acids and increasing inflammation in the process.

Avoid refined carbohydrates: While complex carbohydrates are a great source of energy, refined carbohydrates are typically simple carbohydrates which means they break down extremely quickly while also being responsible for the low energy feeling related to a sugar crash. What"s more, the refining process is simply another word for processing which means they are stripped of what little nutritional value that they would otherwise have. They are also typically high in sugar which makes them a trigger for inflammation in just about every possible way imaginable.

Avoid too much alcohol: When consumed to excess, both beer and hard alcohol have been linked to an increase in inflammation if used regularly. A good rule of thumb is that men should stick with no more than 2 drinks per day and women should limit themselves to 1 drink if they want to drink while at the same time keep their inflammation levels to a minimum.

CHAPTER 2

Breakfast Recipes

Anti-Inflammatory Blueberry Smoothie

Makes enough for: 1

Time required for proper preparation: 5 minutes

Suggested cooking time: 0 minutes

Total required: 5 minutes

What to Use

- Cayenne pepper (.25 tsp.)

- frozen banana (1)

- frozen blueberries (.5 c)

- cinnamon (.25 tsp)

- Maca powder (1 tsp.)

- almond Coconut oil (1 T)

- water (.5)

- spinach or leafy greens (2 handfuls)

- unsweetened almond milk (.5 c)

What to Do

- Add everything to a food processor or blender and blend/process until your desired consistency is reached

Cherry Coconut Porridge

Total required: 15 minutes

What to Use

- Maple syrup (as desired)

- Dark chocolate flakes (as desired)

- Cherries (as desired)

- Coconut shavings (as desired)

- Stevia (1 pinch)

- Cacao (3 T raw)

- Coconut milk (3.5 c)

- Chia seed (4 T)

- Oats (5 c)

What to Do

- In a saucepan, add the stevia, cacao, coconut milk, chia, and oats together before placing the pan on the stove over a burner turned to medium heat.

- Let the mixture boil before turning the heat to low and letting everything simmer until the oats are completely cooked.

- Pour the results into a bowl, add the remaining ingredients as desired and serve hot

Goat Cheese/Zucchini Frittata

Makes enough for: 4

Time required for proper preparation: 10 minutes

Suggested cooking time: 15 minutes

Total required: 25 minutes

What to Use

- Goat cheese (2 oz.)

- Garlic (1 clove)

- Coconut oil (1 T)

- Pepper (as desired)

- Salt (.25 tsp.)

- Milk (2 T)

- Eggs (8)

- Zucchinis (2 sliced)

What to Do

- Ensure your oven is preheated to 350F.

- Combine the pepper, salt, milk, and eggs together in a large bowl.

- Coat a pan in the oil and place it on the stove above a burner that has been turned to a high/medium heat.

- Add in the zucchini and garlic and let them sauté approximately 5 minutes or until done.

- Add in the eggs and stir well for 60 seconds.

- Remove the pan from the stove, top frittata with cheese and bake approximately 11 minutes.

- Let it cool for 3 minutes, serve warm and enjoy.

Tomato Frittata

Makes enough for: 2

Time required for proper preparation: 15 minutes

Suggested cooking time: 10 minutes

Total required: 25 minutes

What to Use

- Halved cherry tomatoes (8)

- Chopped zucchini (1)

- Coconut oil (2 T)

- Pepper

- Salt

- Almond milk (.5 c.)

- Egg whites (3)

- Eggs (3)

- Grated Parmesan cheese (.25 c.)

What to Do

- Heat up the broiler of the oven to high, and move the rack of the oven to the middle.

- Take out a bowl and whisk together the pepper, salt, almond milk, egg whites, and eggs.

- In a skillet, heat up some coconut oil. Let it warm up until it starts to shimmer.

- Add in the tomatoes and the zucchini and cook for about five minutes, stirring a bit.

- Pour in your egg mixture to this and let everything cook for a bit. After four minutes, the edges should start to set.

- Using a spatula, you can pull the eggs away from the pan edges. Tilt the pan around so that the unset egg can make it on all the edges too.

- After another four minutes, you can sprinkle on the Parmesan cheese before transferring the pan to your broiler.

- Cook for three to five minutes so the eggs have time to become puffy. Slice and serve.

Simple Chia Pudding

Makes enough for: 4

Time required for proper preparation: 5 minutes

Suggested cooking time: 6 hours

Total required: 6 hours and 5 minutes

What to Use

- Extract (Vanilla) (1 tsp)

- Agave (1-2 T)

- Dairy-free milk (1.5 c)

- Chia seeds (0.5 c)

What to Do

- First, combine the maple syrup, vanilla extract, chia seeds, and dairy-free milk in a bowl. Then whisk the ingredients very well to mix them all together.

- Refrigerate the ingredients overnight or for at least 6 hours in the bowl (preferably overnight), so the chia pudding is thick and creamy. If the chia pudding is not thick and creamy, you can add more chia seeds. Then put it back into the refrigerator, and keep it in the refrigerator for about another hour or so until the pudding is firm. You can garnish it with fruit, almonds, or nuts of your choice.

Veggie Egg Muffins

Serves: 8

Time required for proper preparation: 20 minutes

Suggested cooking time: 30 minutes

Total required: 50 minutes

What to Use

- Onion (1 small, diced)

- Mushrooms (4 medium, sliced)

- Powdered garlic (2 tsp.)

- Salt (1 tsp.)

- Provolone cheese (.25 c shredded)

- Eggs (8)

- Milk (.25 c)

- Broccoli (2 c cut or torn into small florets)

- Bell pepper (1 c chopped)

What to Do

- Ensure your oven is heated to 350F.

- Grease the muffin pan, and fill with vegetables.

- In a large bowl, add the eggs, garlic powder & salt.

- Fill each c.75of the way with the egg mixture then top with a pinch of cheese.

- Bake approximately 25 to 30 minutes or until puffy and golden brown.

Sweet Potato Breakfast Burrito

Makes enough for: 1

Time required for proper preparation: 25 minutes

Suggested cooking time: 10 minutes

Total required: 35 minutes

What to Use

- Coconut oil (4 tsp.)

- Cheddar cheese (2 oz. shredded)

- Baby spinach (4 c packed, roughly chopped)

- Sweet potatoes (2 small peeled and diced)

- Yellow onions (2 small, chopped)

- Tricolor bell peppers (1.5 c frozen, sliced, thawed)

- 10-inch whole wheat tortillas (8)

- Chili powder (2 tsp.)

- Eggs (4 large beaten)

- Egg whites (4 large, beaten)

What to Do

- Place your skillet on the stove over a burner turned to medium heat. Sauté potato, onion and bell peppers for approximately 7 minutes. Toss in chili powder, spinach, and sauté for another 2 minutes.

- Increase the heat slightly to high/medium. Mix in eggs and egg whites. Cook for 3 minutes, continuing to stir until eggs are cooked completely and not runny. Remove from heat and cool for 10 minutes.

- Cut 8 16-inch pieces of aluminum foil. Place 1 tortilla on top of each piece. Put an equal portion of the egg mixture in the middle of each tortilla. Sprinkle cheese on top. Fold two sides in first, and then roll forward from the top of the burrito. Make sure the foil is wrapped tightly around the burrito, but not inside the roll, if you will be microwaving it to reheat.

- Place burritos into a large plastic bag in the fridge. There are two ways to reheat. You can either bake the burrito on a cookie sheet in a 400-degree oven for 35 minutes or cook in the microwave for 2 minutes. Transfer the burrito to a paper bag with a pair of tongs, and you can bring it with you on the run.

Porridge

Makes enough for: 1

Time required for proper preparation: 5 minutes

Suggested cooking time: 5 minutes

Total required: 10 minutes

What to Use

- Salt (1 pinch)

- Coconut cream (4 T)

- Psyllium husk powder (1 pinch ground)

- Coconut flour (1 T)

- Egg (1)

- Coconut oil (1 oz.)

What to Do

- Place everything together in a small pan before placing the pan on the stove on top of a burner set to low heat.

- Stir the results continuously to encourage porridge to thicken. Continue stirring until your preferred thickness is reached.

- A small amount of coconut milk or a few berries (fresh or frozen) can also be added as desired.

Carrot Muffins

Makes enough for: 12

Time required for proper preparation: 20 minutes

Suggested cooking time: 15 minutes

What to Use

- Ground nutmeg (.5 tsp.)

- Ground ginger (2 tsp.)

- Ground cinnamon (2 tsp.)

- Baking powder (1 tsp.)

- Baking soda (1 tsp.)

- Brown sugar (3 T)

- Old-fashioned oats (.5 c.)

- Whole-wheat flour (1 c.)

- Oat bran (1 c.)

- Cooking spray

- Raisins (.25 c.)

- Grated carrots (1.5 c.)

- Coconut oil (2 T)

- Egg (1)

- Honey (2 T)

- Almond milk (1.25 c.)

- Salt (.25 tsp.)

What to Do

- Ensure your oven is ready at 350F. Line two muffin tins with some paper liners, or use your cooking spray for this.

- Now take out a big bowl and whisk together the salt, nutmeg, ginger, cinnamon, baking powder, baking soda, brown sugar, oats, all the flours, and the oat bran. Set it to the side.

- In another bowl, whisk together the coconut oil, egg, honey, and almond milk.

- Add your dry ingredients and wet ingredients together and mix to just blend. The batter will be lumpy and have some flour streaks still in it, and that is fine.

- Fold in the raisins and the carrots at this time.

- Take the batter and fill up the muffin c before placing into the oven. After 15 minutes, the muffins should be done. Allow them time to cool down before serving.

Berry Smoothie Bowl

Makes enough for: 1

Time required for proper preparation: 5 minutes

Suggested cooking time: 0 minutes

Total required: 5 minutes

What to Use

- Protein powder (1 scoop)

- Almond milk (2-3 T (can substitute coconut milk))

- Sliced ripe banana (1 that is frozen)

- Organic Frozen mixed berries (1 big c)

- Seeds (Hemp and Chia) (1 T)

- Shreds of coconut (Unsweetened) (1 T)

What to Do

- Blend the berries and ripened banana together.

- Add the almond milk to the protein powder and blend both until the mixture is blended smoothly. You can top with chia seeds, hemp seeds, or shredded unsweetened coconut if you would like.

- You can also substitute any non-diary milk if you do not like dairy milk. To take the recipe to another level, you can also substitute a green or white tea as well.

Omelet with Mushrooms

Makes enough for: 1

Time required for proper preparation: 5 minutes

Suggested cooking time: 10 minutes

Total required: 15 minutes

What to Use

- Mushrooms (3 chopped)

- Onion (.25 chopped)

- Sharp cheddar cheese (1 oz. shredded)

- Coconut oil (1 oz. grass fed)

- Pepper (as desired)

- Salt (as desired)

What to Do

- In a mixing bowl, add the eggs and season as desired before whisking well until the eggs become a batter.

- Add in a majority of the onion, mushroom as well as another pinch of salt to the mixing bowl, and mix well.

- Add the coconut oil to a frying pan before placing it on top of a burner set to a high/medium heat. Once the coconut oil is completely melted, add in the batter.

- Once the omelet begins to harden top with the remaining onions and mushrooms before adding the cheese. With the help of a spatula fold the egg on top of itself and continue cooking until it takes on a cooked, golden brown appearance.

Spinach Frittata with Bacon

Makes enough for: 4

Time required for proper preparation: 5 minutes

Suggested cooking time: 35 minutes

Total required: 40 minutes

What to Use

- Pepper (as desired)

- Salt (as desired)

- Coconut oil (2 T grass fed)

- Cheese (5 oz. shredded)

- Bacon (5 oz.)

- Spinach (.5 lbs. fresh)

- Heavy whipping cream (1 c)

- Eggs (8 large)

What to Do

- Start by making sure your oven is heated to 350F.

- Grease a baking dish using grass-fed Coconut oil.

- Add the coconut oil to a frying pan before placing it on the stove on top of a burner set to a medium/high heat before adding in the bacon and letting it fry until it reaches your desired level of crispiness and then add in the spinach.

- Separately, mix together the cream and the eggs before whisking well.

- Add the results to the prepared baking dish before adding in the spinach and the bacon and topping with the shredded cheese.

- Place the dish in the oven for approximately 25 minutes. Let the frittata cool 5 minutes prior to removing from baking dish.

Smoked Salmon Sammie on Pumpkin Bread

This recipe needs 5 minutes to prepare, 10 minutes to cook and will make 2 servings.

Makes enough for: 2

Time required for proper preparation: 5 minutes

Suggested cooking time: 10 minutes

Total required: 15 minutes

What to Use - Bread

- Coconut oil (1 T)
- Pumpkin puree (1 can)
- Coconut oil (.25 c)
- Apple sauce (.5 c unsweetened)
- Eggs (3 large)
- Pumpkin seeds (.3 c)
- Walnuts (.3 c chopped)
- Coconut flour (1.25 c)
- Almond flour (1.25 c)
- Flax seeds (.5 c)
- Psyllium husk (2 T powdered)

- Salt (1 tsp.)

- Baking powder (1 T)

- Pumpkin pie spice (2 T)

What to Use - Filling

- Chives (1 T chopped)

- Salmon (3 oz. smoked)

- Lettuce (1 oz.)

- Coconut oil (2 T grass fed)

- Chili flakes (1 pinch)

- Coconut oil (2 T grass fed)

- Pepper (as desired)

- Salt (as desired)

- Heavy whipping cream (2 T)

- Eggs (4 large)

- Egg (2 scrambled)

What to Do - Bread

- Start by making sure your oven is heated to 400F.

- Grease a bread pan (8 inches) using grass-fed Coconut oil

- In a large bowl add the walnuts, coconut flour, almond flour, flax seeds, psyllium powder, salt, baking powder, and pumpkin pie spice and mix well.

- Mix in the pumpkin puree, coconut oil, apple sauce, and eggs and combine thoroughly.

- Add the batter to the prepared baking dish and top with 1 T pumpkin seeds.

- Place the pan on the bottom rack in the oven and let it bake for 60 minutes. You will know it is finished when you can stick a knife in and it comes out clean.

What to Do - Sammie

- In a small bowl, combine the heavy whipping cream with the eggs and whisk well before seasoning as needed with pepper and salt.

- Add the coconut oil to a frying pan before placing in the stove on top of a burner set to medium heat. Once the coconut oil has melted, add in the egg mixture and stir well prior to removing the frying pan from the stove. Add in the chili powder and mix well

- Add the results to two pieces of toasted pumpkin bread, top with lettuce, smoked salmon, chives and scrambled eggs.

Scrambled Eggs with Avocado and Bacon

Makes enough for: 4

Time required for proper preparation: 2 minutes

Suggested cooking time: 10 minutes

Total required: 12 minutes

What to Use

- Pepper (as desired)

- Salt (as desired)

- Bacon (2 oz.)

- Coconut oil (1 tsp.)

- Avocado (.5 peeled)

- Eggs (2)

What to Do

- Preheat the oven to 350F.

- In a small pot, place the eggs and add cold water until the eggs are completely covered by roughly 1 inch of water. Add the pot to the stove above a boiler turned to a high/medium heat and let the water boil.

- After the water has boiled, remove the pot from the stove, let it cool for roughly 10 minutes, and then drain the pot.

- Fill a large bowl with cold water and dunk the eggs briefly into it to make them easier to peel.

- Peel and prepare the eggs as preferred before placing them in a bowl, they should be warm, not hot.

- Split the eggs, remove the yolks, and discard them.

- In a large bowl, add the eggs, oil, and avocado and mix well before seasoning as desired.

- Place the bacon on a baking sheet and place the baking sheet in the oven approximately 5 minutes or until done.

- Once the bacon is no longer hot to the touch, break each piece in half and portion out a half per serving of eggs.

Ham Omelet with Green Bell Peppers

Makes enough for: 2

Time required for proper preparation: 10 minutes

Suggested cooking time: 15 minutes

Total required: 25 minutes

What to Use

- Ham (5 oz. diced)

- Green bell pepper (.25 chopped fine)

- Onion (.5 yellow chopped fine)

- Coconut oil (2 oz. grass fed)

- Cheese (4 oz. shredded)

- Pepper (as desired)

- Salt (as desired)

- Sour cream (2 T)

- Eggs (6 large)

What to Do

- In a mixing bowl, combine the sour cream and eggs and whisk well before seasoning using salt and pepper as needed. Mix in 2 oz. shredded cheese.

- Add the coconut oil to a frying pan before placing the frying pan on the stove on top of a burner set to medium heat. Add in the onion, green pepper, and ham and let everything cook for 2 minutes or the egg is nearly firm.

- Turn the burner to a low heat before adding the remaining cheese and folding the egg over on top of itself.

Egg Scramble

Makes enough for: 2

Time required for proper preparation: 10 minutes

Suggested cooking time: 15 minutes

Total required: 25 minutes

What to Use

- Pepper (as desired)

- Salt (as desired)

- Coconut oil (2 T)

- Olives (.5 c pitted)

- Parsley (.5 c chopped)

- Scallions (2)

- Halloumi cheese (4 oz. diced)

- Bacon (5 oz. diced)

- 5 eggs (large)

What to Do

- Add the oil to a frying pan before placing the pan on the stove on top of a burner set to medium heat. Add in the bacon, scallions, and halloumi and let it all brown.

- Combine the eggs and parsley in a small bowl and season as desired before whisking.

- Add the results to the pan before reducing the heat, adding in the olives and stir continuously for 2 additional minutes.

Grecian Breakfast Sandwich

Makes enough for: 2

Time required for proper preparation: 5 minutes

Suggested cooking time: 7 minutes

Total required: 12 minutes

What to Use

- Feta cheese (4 T)

- Tomato (1 sliced)

- Baby spinach (2 c)

- Eggs (4)

- Rosemary (1 T)

- Coconut oil (4 T)

- Multigrain sandwich thins (4)

What to Do

- Ensure your oven is preheated to 375F

- Brush the sandwich thins with coconut oil before adding them to a baking sheet and letting them bake approximately 5 minutes or until done.

- Coat a pan in the oil and place it on the stove above a burner that has been turned to a high/medium heat.

- Add the eggs to the pan and let them cook for 60 seconds. Let the yolks break and then flip the eggs and cook for an additional 60 seconds.

- Add all ingredients to sandwich thins, serve warm and enjoy.

Tabbouleh

Makes enough for: 4

Time required for proper preparation: 2 hours

Suggested cooking time: 0 minutes

Total required: 2 hours

What to Use

- Salt and pepper (as desired)
- Cucumber (1 peeled, seeded, chopped)
- Tomatoes (3 chopped)
- Mint (.25 c chopped)
- Parsley (1 c chopped)
- Green onions (1 c chopped)
- Lemon juice (.3 c)
- Coconut oil (.3 c)
- Water (1.5 c boiling)
- Bulgur (1 c)

What to Do

- Add the bulgur to the water, cover the pot and let it sit for 60 minutes.

- Mix in the cucumber, tomatoes, mint, parsley, onions, lemon juice, and oil before seasoning as needed.

- Add the lid back on and let it sit in the refrigerator for at least 60 minutes before serving.

Veggie Cakes

Makes enough for: 2

Time required for proper preparation: 10 minutes

Suggested cooking time: 15 minutes

Total required: 25 minutes

What to Use

- Salt and pepper (as desired)

- Walnuts (2 T chopped)

- Eggs (3 beaten)

- Sun-dried tomatoes (.25 c)

- Almond flour (.3 c)

- Kalamata olives (.3 c, sliced pitted)

- Artichoke hearts (.3 c)

- Parsnip (1 grated)

- Spinach (3 c)

- Garlic (3 cloves chopped)

- Onion (1 c chopped)

- Coconut oil (.25 c divided)

What to Do

- Coat a pan in half the oil and place it on the stove above a burner that has been turned to medium heat.

- Add in the garlic and onion and let them cook approximately 5 minutes or until done.

- Add in the spinach and let it also cook approximately 5 minutes or until done.

- Add the results to a large and let them cool.

- Into the bowl, add the remainder of the ingredients before combining well and forming the results into circles.

- Add the remainder of the oil to the pan and let the circles cook approximately 5 minutes or until done per side.

- Serve hot and enjoy.

Cherry Coconut Porridge

Makes enough for: 1

Time required for proper preparation: 10 minutes

Suggested cooking time: 5 minutes

Total required: 15 minutes

What to Use

- Maple syrup (as desired)
- Dark chocolate flakes (as desired)
- Cherries (as desired)
- Coconut shavings (as desired)
- Stevia (1 pinch)
- Cacao (3 T raw)
- Coconut milk (3.5 c)
- Chia seed (4 T)
- Oats (5 c)

What to Do

- In a saucepan, add the stevia, cacao, coconut milk, chia, and oats together before placing the pan on the stove over a burner turned to medium heat.

- Let the mixture boil before turning the heat to low and letting everything simmer until the oats are completely cooked.

- Pour the results into a bowl, add the remaining ingredients as desired and serve hot.

Ginger, Apple Rhubarb Muffins

Makes enough for: 8

Time required for proper preparation: 15 minutes

Suggested cooking time: 20 minutes

Total required: 35 minutes

What to Use

- Salt (1 pinch)

- Ginger (.5 tsp. ground)

- Cinnamon (.5 tsp. ground)

- Baking powder (2 tsp. gluten-free)

- True arrowroot (2 T)

- Brown rice flour (.25 c)

- Buckwheat flour (.5 c)

- Linseed meal (1 T ground)

- Raw sugar (.25 c)

- Almonds (.5 c ground)

- Vanilla extract (1 tsp.)

- Egg (1 large)

- Coconut oil (.25 c)

- Rice milk (.3 c, 1 T)

- Apple (1 peeled, cored, diced)

- Rhubarb (1 c sliced)

What to Do

- Ensure your oven is heated to 350F.

- Coat a muffin tin in baking spray and add muffin liners.

- In a medium-sized bowl, mix together the linseed meal, ginger, sugar and almond meal.

- Mix the spices, flours and baking powder in evenly before adding the apple and rhubarb.

- In a separate bowl, add vanilla, egg, oil, and milk together before adding the results to the initial bowl.

- Add the batter to the tin, place the tin in the oven and let the muffins cook for 22 minutes. You will know they are finished when you can stick a toothpick into one of the muffins and it comes out dry.

- Let the muffins cool before serving.

CHAPTER 3

Vegetarian Recipes

<u>Hearts of Palm Black Bean Salad</u>

Makes enough for: 2

Time required for proper preparation: 10 minutes

Suggested cooking time: 0 minutes

Total required: 10 minutes

What to Use

- Coconut oil (3 T)

- Vinegar (2 T)

- Parsley leaves (1 tsp fresh cut into small pieces)

- Jalapeño pepper (1 take out the seeds before using)

- Cilantro leaves (1 T cut into small pieces)

- Hearts of Palm (1 can)

- Lime juice (2 T)

- Chives (1 tsp fresh, cut into small pieces)

- Red onion (1 cut into thin slices)

- Black beans (1 c cooked according to package)

- Green onions (1 T)

- Corn (1 c cooked according to package)

- Yellow pepper (.5 c cut into thin slices)

- Avocado, (1 cut into small cubes)

- Pepper (as desired)

- Salt (as desired)

What to Do

- Using a mixing bowl, thoroughly combine vinegar, coconut oil, herbs, jalapeño, lime juice, salt, and Black pepper (as desired). Put to the side while preparing the salad.

- Cut the hearts of palm into.5 inch slices, making sure to cut at an angle.

- In another mixing bowl, mix the hearts of palm, black beans, red onions, corn, bell pepper, and green onions.

- When using for an appetizer, the mix can be served over greens. Add dressing over salad, top with avocado.

Makes enough for: 6

Time required for proper preparation: 10 minutes

Suggested cooking time: 1 hour 35 minutes

Total required: 1 hour 45 minutes

What to Use

- Spaghetti squash (1 large, ripe)

- Salt (as desired)

- Pepper (as desired)

- Marinara sauce (2 c)

- Ricotta (1 c)

- Parmesan cheese (8 tsp.)

- Mozzarella (6 oz. shredded)

What to Do

- Preheat oven to 375F.

- Cut the squash in half, and scoop out all the seeds and fibers with a spoon.

- Place on a baking sheet, with the cut side up, and season with the salt and pepper.

- Bake at 375F about an hour or until the skin gives easily under pressure and the inside is tender. Remove from oven and let it cool for 10 minutes.

- Use a fork to create "noodles" from the squash. It will fluff up into spaghetti-like strands.

- Pour.25 c quick marinara sauce on the bottom of four individual 5 x 7-inch pans. Top the sauce with.75c of the spaghetti squash and spread evenly. Add.25 the total ricotta to each, top with mozzarella. Add mozzarella and bake approximately 11 minutes.

Root Vegetable Casserole

Makes enough for: 4

Time required for proper preparation: 30 minutes

Suggested cooking time: 1 hour 30 minutes

Total required: 2 hours

What to Use

- Coconut oil (as needed)

- Heavy cream (1 c)

- Sour cream (6 T)

- Whole milk (1 c)

- Black pepper(as desired)

- Sea salt (as desired)

- Cheddar cheese (6 oz. grated)

- Celeriac (11 oz. halved, peeled, sliced thin)

- Turnips (13 oz. halved, peeled, sliced thin)

- Potatoes (1.5 lbs. halved, peeled, sliced thin)

- Rutabaga (1 lb. halved, peeled, sliced thin)

What to Do

- Ensure your oven is heated to 400F. Cover a baking dish (8x12) in coconut oil

- In a mixing bowl, combine the slices of celeriac, turnip, potatoes, and rutabaga together and mix well

- Place a saucepan on the stove on top of a burner set to a low heat before adding in the milk, sour cream and regular cream and mix until combined. Remove the saucepan from the burner and season using pepper as well as salt and stir repeatedly.

- Place half of the total amount of sliced root vegetables into a baking dish before seasoning and topping with a third of all of the cheese. Add a third of the total cream mixture to the top of the vegetables before adding in the rest of the vegetables and the rest of the cheese. Top with the rest of the cream.

- Place the results in the oven and let them bake for 90 minutes until the top is well-browned. Allow to cool and portion out into containers or plastic bags. This recipe can be refrigerated for 3-4 days or frozen for 2-3 months.

Enchiladas

Makes enough for: 6

Time required for proper preparation: 30 minutes

Suggested cooking time: 30 minutes

Total required: 1 hour

What to Use

- Water (3.5 c)

- Lime juice (1 T)

- Vegetable broth (.5 c low sodium, fat-free)

- Black beans (.6 c drained and rinsed)

- Tomato paste (1 T low-sodium)

- Kosher sea salt (as desired)

- Cumin (.5 tsp. ground)

- Mexican style crema (6 T)

- Onions (3 divided, sliced)

- Monterey Jack cheese (2 oz. shredded)

- Cheddar cheese (2.5 oz. shredded)

- Corn tortillas (12)

- Oregano (1 tsp.)

267

- Garlic (4 tsp. minced)

- Onion (2 c chopped)

- Coconut oil (2 tsp.)

- Enchilada sauce (28 oz. can red or green)

What to Do

- Preheat oven to 400F.

- Place a skillet on top of a stove over a burner set to medium heat. Place oil in the pan; swirl to coat. Add onion; cook until tender, stirring as needed

- Add garlic, oregano, cumin, and salt and let it cook 2 minutes while still stirring before adding in the tomato paste and letting everything cook an additional minute.

- Add in the broth, beans, and beef and let everything cook another minute, still stirring. After you have removed it from heat, add in the lime juice.

- Wrap six tortillas at a time in a wet paper towel covering the top and the bottom. Microwave for 45 seconds or until soft. In each tortilla, at 3 T of the beef before rolling tightly.

- Add half a cup of the sauce to the bottom of a glass baking dish (13 x 9) that has been prepared using cooking spray before placing the enchiladas into the dish. Pour remaining enchilada sauce over the enchiladas. Top with the cheeses.

- Add the dish to the oven and let it bake at 400F for approximately 20 minutes. You are looking for it to be lightly browned and bubbly. Let the enchiladas stand 10 minutes. Top with the green onions and crema if serving immediately. This makes a great frozen dish.

Black Bean and Red Pepper Quinoa Salad

Makes enough for: 4

Time required for proper preparation: 10 minutes

Suggested cooking time: 15 minutes

Time total: 25 minutes

What to Use - Salad

- Quinoa (.75 c)

- Water (1.5 c)

- Salt (1 pinch)

- Green onion (.3 c thinly sliced)

- Red bell pepper (1 chopped)

- Cilantro (.5 c chopped)

- Black beans (1 can drained, rinsed)

What to Use - Dressing

- Lime juice (2 T)

- Seasoning salt (1 tsp.)

- Black pepper (as desired)

- Cumin (1 tsp. ground)

- Coconut oil (.25 c)

- Paprika or other chili powder (.5 tsp.)

What to Do

- Rinse the quinoa using a strainer before adding it, the salt and the water to a pot before placing it on the stove over a burner turned to high heat. Once it boils, turn the heat down and allow it to simmer while covered until all the water has been completely absorbed. Fluff the quinoa and set aside.

- Drain the beans into a colander in the sink and rinse with cold water, until all the foam is gone. Drain beans until they are very dry (or pat with paper towels to speed it up.)

- Once the quinoa has cooled, add in the non-dressing ingredients and mix well. Portion it out into 8 containers and sprinkle some chopped cilantro on top. You can mix in the dressing right away or keep the dressing on the side and add in a little before eating. This meal will remain good for 3 days as long as it is refrigerated.

Asparagus and Farro Salad

Serves: 4

Time required for proper preparation: 20 minutes

Suggested cooking time: 30 minutes

Total required: 50 minutes

What to Use - Salad

- Farro (1 c)

- Asparagus (1 c sliced)

- Coconut oil (3 tsp.)

- Lemon juice (1 tsp.)

- Green onions (.6 c sliced)

- Parsley (.5 c chopped)

- Red pepper (1 diced)

What to Use - Dressing

- Capers (.3 c juice included)

- Sun-dried tomatoes (3 T chopped)

- Parsley (2 T chopped)

- Red wine vinegar (.3 c)

- Coconut oil (.3 c)

- Lemon juice (2 tsp.)

- Dijon mustard (1 tsp.)

What to Do

- Add the farro to a skillet before placing the skillet on the stove on top of a high/medium heat until it begins to brown. You will then want to turn off the heat before adding in 1.75 c boiling water to the skillet, as well as a pinch of salt. Turn the burner to low and let it cook for 20 minutes. Add a small amount of water if necessary.) Drain excess water.

- As the farro cooks, you will want to add the parsley, tomatoes, and capers to your food processor or blender and go nuts well. Add the pureed results into a bowl before adding in the red wine vinegar, Dijon and lemon juice before adding in the coconut oil and whisking well.

- After the farro has cooled, add it to a separate bowl and add.25 c of the previous bowl into this one.

- Add 2 tsp. coconut oil in a heavy pan, and sauté asparagus slices approximately 5 minutes or until done. Add in the remainder of the lemon juice and add the results to the bowl of farro

- Add the oil to the pan before placing it on top of a burner turned to a high/medium heat. Add in the red pepper and allow it to sauté about 1 minute before adding it to the farro mixture and combining thoroughly.

- Add the chopped parsley and sliced green onions together in a bowl and mix well. Add dressing to your liking or keep on the side to add before serving. This will keep for 3 days in the fridge.

Black Bean Stew

Serves: 6

Time required for proper preparation: 15 minutes

Suggested cooking time: 75 minutes

Total required: 1 hour 30 minutes

What to Use

- Coconut oil (2 T)

- White onion (1 large diced)

- Black beans (7 c cooked, drained)

- Plum tomatoes (28 oz. diced)

- Cilantro stems (.25 c chopped, leaves reserved for serving)

- Kosher salt (2 tsp. more as needed)

- Scallion (1 sliced, for serving)

- Lime wedges (for serving)

- Diced avocado (for serving)

What to Do

- Place the oil in a heavy pot before placing the pot on the stove on top of a burner set to medium heat. Add onion and cook, stirring occasionally, until softened, 5 to 10 minutes. Add in the cilantro stems and cook an additional 5 minutes over high heat.

- Stir in beans, tomatoes and their juices, and the water. Let the results boil, before reducing to medium.

- Cover the pot partially and simmer until tomatoes fall apart, between 1 hour and 1 hour 15 minutes. Top with avocado, scallion, cilantro leaves and lime wedges to serve.

Lentil Chili and Cornbread

Makes enough for: 6

Time required for proper preparation: 10 minutes

Suggested cooking time: 55 minutes

Total required: 65 minutes

What to Use

- Dry lentils (1.25 c)

- Coconut oil (2 T)

- Water (4 c)

- Onion (1 or 2 T minced)

- Vegetable broth (3 c)

- Tomatoes (15 oz. can)

- Garlic (1 clove minced)

- Chili powder (1.75 tsp.)

- Salt (.25 tsp.)

- Cayenne pepper (1 tsp.)

- Black pepper (as desired)

- Paprika (1 tsp.)

What to Do

- Prepare the lentils by rinsing them and sorting them before adding them in a pot along with the vegetable broth and water before placing the pot on the stove over a burner set to a high heat until it boils.

- Turn down the heat and let the pot simmer, covered, for half an hour.

- After the lentils have fully cooked, add in the rest of the ingredients and let everything simmer 25 more minutes.

Garbanzo Bean Soup

Makes enough for: 8

Time required for proper preparation: 15 minutes

Suggested cooking time: 22 minutes

Total required: 37 minutes

What to Use

- Coconut oil
- Garlic (1 clove minced)
- Garbanzo beans (2 c cooked)
- Potato (1 diced)
- Vegetable broth (3 c)
- Salt (as desired)
- Pepper (as desired)
- Thyme (.3 tsp. dried)
- Carrot (1)
- Bay leaf (1)
- Onion (. 3 diced)
- Celery (1 stalk diced)

What to Do

- Start by sautéing the thyme, onion, celery, carrot and bay leaf on medium heat in a drizzle of oil.

- Wait 10 minutes before adding in the chickpeas, garlic, and potato and letting it all cook 2 minutes.

- Mix in the broth before allowing it to simmer for 20 minutes and seasoning as desired.

- At this point, you may choose to leave the soup chunky or make it smooth with an immersion or stand-up blender.

Herbed Balsamic Lentils with Polenta

Makes enough for: 4

Time required for proper preparation: 10 minutes

Suggested cooking time: 30 minutes

Total required: 40 minutes

What to Use

- Water (4 c)

- Onion (1 c diced)

- Carrots (2 c)

- Celery (1 c chopped)

- Garlic (4 T)

- Tomato paste (2 T)

- Oregano (.3 tsp. dried)

- Thyme (.3 tsp. dried)

- Brown lentils (.6c)

- Vegetable broth (5 c)

- Black pepper (1 tsp)

- Coconut oil (1 T)

- Salt (1 tsp.)

- Coconut oil (4 T)

- Cornmeal (.75 c)

- Pepper (1 tsp.)

What to Do

- Add the celery, onion, and carrots to a skillet set to a medium/high heat and let them sauté in Coconut oil for 2 minutes.

- After a few minutes, mix in the oregano, thyme, garlic and tomato paste.

- Cook the dry spices and garlic for another minute before adding the lentils.

- Heat them through and then add the broth to the vegetable and lentil mixture. Cover and cook 25 minutes.

- While the lentils are cooking, you"ll prepare the polenta.

- Finish the lentils with balsamic vinegar and salt and pepper as desired. Serve over cheesy polenta.

Curried Lentilsand Rice

Makes enough for: 6

Time required for proper preparation: 10 minutes

Suggested cooking time: 1 hour

Total required: 1 hour and 10 minutes

What to Use

- Vegetable broth (1 - 2 T)

- Granny Smith apple (1 diced)

- Onion (.3 chopped)

- Currants (.3 c)

- Curry powder (3 tsp.)

- Ginger (.3 tsp. ground)

- Vegetable bouillon cubes (3)

- Turmeric (.3 tsp.)

- Water (3.5 c)

- Lentils (.5 c dried)

- Brown rice (.75 c)

What to Do

- Add the broth to a soup pot before using it to sauté the 1 clove of garlic and the onion.

- Mix in the ginger, turmeric and curry powder and let everything cook for 2 minutes before adding in the rice and letting everything cook 2 minutes more, then adding in the rest of the ingredients except for the apples.

- Increase the heat until the pot boils before turning the heat back down and letting everything simmer about half an hour. Add in the apples and simmer for another half an hour.

- Serve with a dollop of yogurt.

Japanese Red Bean Soup with Spinach Recipe

Makes enough for: 4

Time required for proper preparation: 15 minutes

Suggested cooking time: 35 minutes

Total required: 50 minutes

What to Use

- Red beans (.5 c soaked in water 4 hours or more)
- Bay leaf (1)
- Water (1.5 c)
- Onion (1 large, chopped)
- Carrots (2 cut into small slices)
- Celery (1 stalk cut into small slices)
- Shitake mushrooms (1 c cut into small slices)
- Coconut oil (1 T)
- Garlic (3 cloves cut into tiny pieces)
- Ginger (2 T grated)
- Vegetable stock (4 c)
- Sea salt (as desired)

- Thyme (1 tsp.)

- Cayenne pepper (as desired)

- Spinach (2 c chopped)

- Scallions (2 thinly sliced)

What to Do

- Remove the water from the beans. Place the beans, Kombu, bay leaf and water in a medium-sized pan. Bring water to a boil. Cover the pan and allow to simmer for approximately 1 hour or until just about tender.

- Turn the stove to low/medium, then in a large pot, add coconut oil. Mix in onions, carrots, celery, and sauté until soft and tender, for approximately 5 minutes.

- Add in the mushrooms, continue sautéing for approximately 5 minutes until mushrooms begin to soften and become golden.

- Mix in the ginger and garlic, cooking for about 1 minute.

- Without removing the liquid from the beans, add them in, as well as the stock, thyme, salt and cayenne as desired.

- Continue simmering for another 25 minutes, stirring every so often.

- When the beans and mushrooms are soft and tender, add in the spinach. Stir until the spinach has wilted

- Taste to adjust seasoning as desired.

- Serve the dish with the scallions as a garnish.

Sweet Potato Burgers

Up to 50 minutes prep, 30 minutes for setting, 8 minutes cook time. Makes about six servings.

Makes enough for: 6

Time required for proper preparation: 50 minutes

Suggested cooking time: 10 minutes

Total required: 60 minutes

What to Use

- Quinoa (1.5 c cooked)

- Black beans (1 15-oz. can drained, rinsed)

- Sweet potato (1 large peeled, cubed)

- Red onion (.5 c diced)

- Garlic (2 cloves minced)

- Cilantro (.5 c + 2 T chopped)

- Jalapeno (5 medium, diced, seed removed)

- Cumin (1 tsp. ground)

- Cajun seasoning (2 tsp.)

- Oat Flour (.25 c)

- Salt (as desired)

- Pepper (as desired)

- Coconut oil (2 T)

- Sprouts (as desired)

- Bib lettuce (6 leaves)

- Avocado (.5 large, diced)

- Plain Greek yogurt (.25 c)

- Lime juice (1 tsp.)

- Hot sauce (as desired)

What to Do

- Cook the sweet potatoes for about four minutes or until soft. If roasting the potatoes, place them on a baking tray in an oven pre-heated to 400F. Roast them for about 30 minutes. Remove the skins when cooked.

- Place the sweet potatoes into a blender. Add the black beans, Cajun seasoning, cumin, garlic, cilantro, and red onion and blend until smooth.

- In a large mixing bowl, transfer the blender ingredients in with the cooked quinoa. Stir together until combined. Season as desired

- Stir in the flour to thicken the mixture. You may not need the entire amount.

- Form the mixture into six "burgers," using about .5 c of the mixture for each patty. Place on parchment paper and cool them in the fridge for about 30 minutes.

- While cooling, make the avocado cream. In the blender or food processor, add the avocado, lime juice, and remaining cilantro. Pulse until creamy. Add to the fridge to cool with the patties.

- When ready to cook, warm coconut oil in a large skillet over high/medium heat. Place the "burgers" into the skillet and cook for about four minutes on each side. Serve with the cream on top when done.

Quesadilla and Avocado Salsa

Makes enough for: 4

Time required for proper preparation: 25 minutes

Suggested cooking time: 20 minutes

Total required: 45 minutes

What to Use

- Gluten-free tortillas (4)
- Monterey Jack cheese (1 c shredded)
- Baby spinach leaves (2 c lightly packed)
- Green chills (4 oz. diced)
- Avocado (1 smashed)
- Jalapeño peppers (1 or 2 seeded, halved)
- Lime juice (2 T)
- Coconut oil (2 T)
- Parmesan cheese (2 T)
- Garlic (1 clove)
- Salt (.5 tsp.)
- Cilantro (1 c)

What to Do

- Add all avocado sauce ingredients to a blender or food processor and blend until smooth.

- Place a skillet on top of the stove over a burner set to a medium heat before adding in a tortilla, 1 T green chilies,.25 c of cheese and.5 c spinach.

- Fold the results in half and let it cook for 2 minutes per side, repeat until all the ingredients have been used.

- Slice up the quesadillas and serve with the avocado sauce. They can be wrapped in foil and refrigerated for 3-4 days or frozen for 2-3 months. Reheat in a toaster oven for best results.

Poached Egg and Curry Potatoes

Makes enough for: 4

Time required for proper preparation: 10 minutes

Suggested cooking time: 30 minutes

Total required: 40 minutes

What to Use

- Potato, russet (2 large cubed)

- Ginger (1 in. nub peeled, minced)

- Garlic (2 cloves minced)

- Coconut oil (1 T)

- Curry powder (2 T)

- Tomato sauce (15 oz.)

- Eggs (4 large)

- Cilantro (.5 bunch chopped)

What to Do

- Warm water in a large stockpot and add the potatoes. Cover and boil on high heat for about five minutes. Drain and set aside.

- Warm the oil in a large skillet over low/medium heat. Add the garlic and ginger and cook for about two minutes. Stir in the curry powder and cook for another minute.

- Pour in the tomato sauce into the skillet and mix well. Increase the heat to medium and warm. Add salt if desired.

- Carefully add the potatoes, taking care not to splash the sauce. Mix to cover the potatoes. Add a bit of water to the skillet if the sauce is too thick.

- Push the sauce and potatoes aside, creating four wells to add the eggs. Crack each egg into the skillet. Cover and cook for about ten minutes or until eggs are well-cooked. Sprinkle cilantro on top, if desired.

CHAPTER 4

Seafood Recipes

Fish Sandwich

Makes enough for: 4

Time required for proper preparation: 10 minutes

Suggested cooking time: 10 minutes

Total required: 20 minutes

What to Use

- Salmon fillet (1 lb. quartered)

- Cajun seasoning (2 tsp.)

- Avocado (1 pitted, peeled)

- Mayonnaise (2 T)

- Wheat rolls (4)

- Arugula (1 c)

- Plum tomatoes (2 sliced thin)

- Red onion (.5 c sliced thin)

- Coconut oil (2 T)

What to Do

- Coat the grill in coconut oil before ensuring it is heated to high heat.

- Coat the fish using the seasoning before adding it to the grill and let it cook for approximately 3 minutes on each side.

- Mash the avocado before mixing it with the mayonnaise and spreading on the rolls prior to serving.

- Season as required, serve hot and enjoy.

Sardine Casserole

Makes enough for: 4

Time required for proper preparation: 15 minutes

Suggested cooking time: 40 minutes

Total required: 55 minutes

What to Use

- Bread crumbs (2 T)

- Basil (1 T)

- Garlic (2 cloves chopped)

- Cherry tomatoes (.5 lbs. diced)

- Sardines (17.5 oz.)

- Coconut oil (3 T)

- Russet potatoes (1 lb.)

What to Do

- Add the potatoes to a pot before covering them with salted water and letting the pot boil.

- Once it boils, turn the heat to low/medium before placing a lid on it and letting the potatoes cook for 20 minutes.

- Drain the potatoes and cover them in cold water to let them cool.

- Slice and peel the potatoes.

- Ensure your oven is heated to 350F.

- Add the coconut oil to a casserole dish and coat well.

- Alternate layers of potato and layers of sardine, adding the tomatoes to the sardine layers. Top with bread crumbs, basil, and garlic.

- Let the casserole cook for 20 minutes, serve hot and enjoy.

Mexican Salad with Mahi-Mahi

Makes enough for: 4

Time required for proper preparation: 75 minutes

Suggested cooking time: 20 minutes

Total required: 95 minutes

What to Use

- Ground beef (1 lb.)

- Pepper (as desired)

- Salt (as desired)

- Hot pepper sauce (as desired)

- Chili powder (.5 tsp.)

- Cumin (.5 T ground)

- Cilantro (.25 c chopped)

- Garlic (1 clove crushed)

- Agave sweetener (2 T)

- Lemon juice (1 T)

- Lime juice (2 T)

- Red wine vinegar (.5 c)

- Coconut oil (.5 c)

- Red onion (1 chopped)

- Corn kernels (10 oz. frozen)

- Red bell pepper (1 chopped)

- Green bell pepper (1 chopped)

- Cannellini beans (15 oz. rinsed, drained)

- Kidney beans (15 oz. rinsed, drained)

- Black beans (15 oz. drained, rinsed)

- Mahi-mahi (32 oz.)

What to Do

- In a serving bowl, combine the red onion, frozen corn, bell peppers, and beans and mix well.

- In a smaller separate bowl combine the pepper, cumin, cilantro, hot pepper sauce, garlic, salt, sugar, lemon juice, lime juice, red wine vinegar and coconut oil and whisk well.

- Pour the dressing over the salad and toss well to coat, cover the salad with plastic wrap and allow it to chill in the refrigerator and serve chilled.

- Prior to serving Season the fish as desired.

- Add the coconut oil to a pan before placing the pan on the stove over a burner set to medium heat.

- Add in the fish and let it cook for approximately 5 minutes on each side.

Flounder with Capers, Olives, and Tomatoes

This recipe needs 20 minutes to prepare, 20 minutes to cook and will make 4 servings.

Makes enough for: 4

Time required for proper preparation: 20 minutes

Suggested cooking time: 20 minutes

Total required: 40 minutes

What to Use

- Pepper (as desired)

- Extra virgin coconut oil (2 T)

- Basil (6 leaves torn)

- Flounder (1 lb. fillets)

- Parmesan cheese (3 T grated)

- Basil (6 leaves chopped)

- Lemon juice (1 tsp. fresh)

- Capers (.25 c)

- White wine (.25 c)

- Kalamata olives (24 chopped, pitted)

- Italian seasoning (1 pinch)

- Garlic (2 cloves chopped)

- Spanish onion (.5 chopped)

- Tomatoes (5 rinsed)

What to Do

- Ensure your oven is heated to 425F.

- Fill a saucepan with water and a pinch of salt before placing it on the stove on top of a burner that has been turned to high heat. Once the water boils, add in the tomatoes before pulling them right back out again. Ensure you have a bowl of cold water ready to add them to. Once they are cool enough to handle, remove the skin prior to chopping.

- Add the coconut oil to the skillet before placing the skillet on the stove on top of a burner set to medium heat. Add in the onion and let it cook approximately 5 minutes until it is tender. Add in the Italian seasoning, garlic, and tomatoes and let everything cook about 6 minutes.

- Add in half of the basil, the lemon juice, capers, wine, and olives before turning the heat down and mixing in the parmesan cheese. Let everything cook approximately 15 minutes and it has formed a thick sauce.

- Add the flounder to a baking dish before topping with sauce and basil leaves.

- Place the dish in the oven and let it cook about 10 minutes until the flesh of the fish can easily be flaked with a fork.

Artichokes with Baked Cod

Makes enough for: 2

Time required for proper preparation: 20 minutes

Suggested cooking time: 15 minutes

Total required: 35 minutes

What to Use

- Red onion (.5 wedged)

- Zucchini (2 sliced)

- Garlic clove (1 minced)

- Thyme leaves (2 tsp.)

- Parsley (1 T chopped)

- Black pepper(as desired)

- Cod fillet (2, 6 oz.)

- Lemon juice (2 T)

- Lemon zest (2 T)

- Kalamata olives (8 pitted, chopped)

- Artichoke hearts (14 0z. can)

- Extra virgin coconut oil (1 T)

What to Do

- Ensure your oven has been heated to 450F.

- Coat a pan in the oil and place it on the stove above a burner that has been turned to a high/medium heat.

- Add the onions, thyme, garlic, and zucchini to the pan and let them sauté, you will be able to tell when they are finished because the onions will be practically see through.

- Remove the pan from the burner and mix in the zest, lemon juice, olives, and artichoke hearts.

- Season fish as desired before adding it to the pan and placing the pan in the oven for 15 minutes until the center of the fish is no longer see through.

- Top with parsley prior to serving.

Makes enough for: 3

Time required for proper preparation: 120 minutes

Suggested cooking time: 10 minutes

Total required: 130 minutes

What to Use

- Salmon (5 oz.)

- Cilantro (1 T)

- Purple or yellow onion (.25 c)

- Black pepper (.25 tsp.)

- Fresh lemon juice (3 T)

- Coconut oil (2 T)

What to Do

- Chop the onion and the cilantro.

- Mix the cilantro, onion, black pepper and blend with the tuna.

- Mix in lemon juice.

- Cover and place in refrigerator to marinate for at least 2 hours.

- Add the coconut oil to a pan before placing the pan on the stove over a burner set to medium heat.

- Add in the fish and let it cook for approximately 5 minutes on each side

Tuna Salad

Makes enough for: 1

Time required for proper preparation: 10 minutes

Suggested cooking time: 0 minutes

Total required: 10 minutes

What to Use

- Pine nuts (2 T)

- Orange (1 segmented)

- Basil (2 T chopped)

- Wild Mushrooms (2.5 oz. sliced)

- Romaine lettuce (5 oz. torn)

- Extra virgin coconut oil (.5 T)

- Black pepper(as desired)

- Lemon juice (1 T +.5 tsp. lemon juice)

- Hummus (3 T)

- Green onion (1.5 oz. chopped)

- Celery (1.75 oz. chopped)

- Tuna (6 oz.)

What to Do

- Combine the pepper, the T of lemon juice, hummus, green onion, celery, and tuna together in a small bowl and stir together well.

- In a separate bowl, combine the remaining lemon juice and the extra virgin coconut oil before adding in half of the basil as well as the mushrooms and lettuce.

- Combine the two bowls and mix well before topping with the basil and the pine nuts.

Avocado and Tuna Lettuce Wrap

Makes enough for: 1

Time required for proper preparation: 5 minutes

Suggested cooking time: 0 minutes

Total required: 5 minutes

What to Use

- lettuce leaves (2 large)

- Tuna (8 oz.)

- Avocado (.5)

- Paleo mayo (2 T)

- Green olives (.25 c pitted, sliced)

- Pepper (as desired)

- Salt (as desired)

- Green chilies (2 T diced)

What to Do

- Chop the olives, scallion and green chilies before adding them to a mixing bowl. Mash the avocado before adding it in as well. The avocado should have a texture that appears creamy.

- Add in the mayonnaise as well as the tuna and mix well

- Add the results from the mixing bowl to the lettuce leaves, splitting the tuna in half.

- Roll like a burrito, serve and enjoy.

Tuna Panini

Makes enough for: 4

Time required for proper preparation: 10 minutes Suggested cooking time: 15 minutes

Total required: 25 minutes

What to Use

- Coconut oil (2 tsp.)

- Salt (as desired)

- Black pepper (as desired)

- Wholegrain bread (8 slices)

- Lemon juice (1 tsp.)

- Capers (1 tsp. chopped)

- Kalamata olives (1 T chopped, pitted)

- Red onion (2 T minced)

- Artichoke hearts (2 T chopped)

- Feta cheese (.25 c crumbled)

- Plum tomato (1 chopped)

- Light tuna (12 oz. chunked)

What to Do

- Flake the tuna in a bowl with the help of a fork. Mix in the pepper, salt, lemon juice, capers, olives, onion, artichokes, feta, and tomato and combine well.

- Place.5 c of the tuna mixture on half of the slices. And top the sandwiches.

- Add the oil to a skillet and place the skillet on the stove over a burner set to a high/medium heat. Add 2 panini to the skillet at a time, and cook the first side for 2 minutes, turn the heat down to low/medium and cook the other side for 2 minutes.

- Add additional oil for the second set of sandwiches as needed.

Sweet Potatoes, Tuna, and Capers

Makes enough for: 2

Time required for proper preparation: 10 minutes

Suggested cooking time: 30 minutes

Total required: 40 minutes

What to Use

- Salt (as desired)

- Pepper (as desired)

- Capers (1 T)

- Green onion (1 cut into rings)

- Greek yogurt (2 T)

- Coconut oil (.5 T)

- Chili powder (1 T)

- Tuna (8 oz.)

- Sweet Potatoes (4)

What to Do

- Ensure your air fryer is set to 320F.

- Soak the potatoes for half an hour before drying them and covering them using the coconut oil.

- Place them in the basket, place the basket in the air fryer and let the potatoes cook for 30 minutes.

- While the potatoes are cooking, combine the chili powder, yogurt, and tuna in a bowl before adding pepper, salt and half of the ringed green onion.

- Slice the potatoes in half and hallow them out enough to add in the tuna mixture, capers, and the remaining green onion.

Yellow Fin Tuna with Poke

Makes enough for: 2

Time required for proper preparation: 5 minutes

Suggested cooking time: 10 minutes

Total required: 15 minutes

What to Use

- Salt (as desired)

- Pepper (as desired)

- Red grapefruit (.25)

- Pili nuts (.25 c)

- Sesame seeds (1 T)

- Sesame oil (2 T)

- Avocado (.5)

- Cilantro (5 sprigs)

- Coconut aminos (1 T)

- Tuna (8 oz. grilled)

What to Do

- Slice the tuna into .25 in. cubes and add to a large mixing bowl before mixing in the salt, pepper, sesame oil and coconut aminos and toss gently.

- Add in the grapefruit, pili nuts, avocado, and cilantro and mix well.

- Divide the results into two bowls and top with sesame seeds prior to serving.

Cheesy Tuna Casserole

Makes enough for: 4

Time required for proper preparation: 10 minutes

Suggested cooking time: 15 minutes

Total required: 25 minutes

What to Use

- Tuna (two 6-oz. cans, drained)

- Green beans (16-oz. bag, French-cut, frozen)

- Mushrooms (3 oz., fresh, sliced)

- Coconut oil (2 T)

- Chicken broth (.5 c)

- Heavy cream (.75 c)

- Onion (2 T chopped fine)

- Salt and pepper (as desired)

- Xanthan gum (optional)

- Celery (1 stalk, hashed fine)

- Cheddar cheese (4-8 oz., shredded)

What to Do

- Cook the green beans in a medium pot. Drain well.

- Place the coconut oil, celery, mushrooms, and onion in a pan and place the pan on top of the stove over a burner turned to medium heat and let everything cook approximately 5 minutes or until done.

- Add the broth. Boil, letting the liquid cook down by half.

- Stir in the cream. Let come back up to a boil.

- Turn down the heat until the sauce is thickened, stirring frequently. Don"t let it boil over.

- Season as desired.

- Put the mushroom mixture and tuna into the green beans.

- Add salt and pepper if needed.

- Put the cheese in it, thoroughly mixing it in.

- Put the mixture into a 1.5 or 2-quart casserole dish.

- Microwave or bake until hot.

Caper Salad with a Mediterranean Twist

Makes enough for: 4

Time required for proper preparation: 10 minutes

Suggested cooking time: 0 minutes

Total required: 10 minutes

What to Use

- Tomatoes (2 large)
- Pepper (as desired)
- Salt (as desired)
- Lemon juice (1 T)
- Capers (1 T)
- Basil (2 T)
- Red peppers (2 T roasted, chopped)
- Red onion (2 T minced)
- Kalamata olives (.25 c chopped)
- Mayonnaise (.25 c)
- Tuna (10 oz.)

What to Do

- In a large bowl, mix everything, save the tomatoes together.

- Cut the tops of the tomatoes off, remove the insides, add the tuna mixture to the tomatoes, serve and enjoy.

Fish Soup

Makes enough for: 6

Time required for proper preparation: 15 minutes

Suggested cooking time: 4 hours and 20 minutes

Total required: 4 hours and 35 minutes

What to Use

- Cod (1 lb. cubed)

- Shrimp (1 lb. deveined, peeled)

- Salt and pepper (as desired)

- Fennel seed (.25 tsp. crushed)

- Basil (1 tsp.)

- Bay leaves (2)

- Dry white wine (.5 c)

- Orange juice (.5 c)

- Black olives (.25 c sliced)

- Mushrooms (2.5 oz.)

- Tomato sauce (8 oz.)

- Chicken broth (28 oz.)

- Tomatoes (14.5 oz. can diced, drained)

- Garlic (2 cloves minced)

- Bell pepper (.5 chopped)

- Onion (1 chopped)

What to Do

- Add the pepper, fennel, basil, bay, wine, juice, olives, mushroom, tomato sauce, chicken broth, tomatoes, garlic, bell pepper, and onion into a crockpot, cover it and let everything cook on a low temperature for 4 hours.

- Add in the cod as well as the shrimp, return the lid to the crockpot and let it cook until the shrimp turn opaque which should take 20 minutes.

- Serve hot and enjoy.

Fish Cakes

Makes enough for: 4

Time required for proper preparation: 2 hours and 30 minutes

Suggested cooking time: 10 minutes

Total required: 2 hours and 40 minutes

What to Use

- Whole wheat flour (4 T)
- Shrimp (6.5 oz.)
- Tuna (9 oz.)
- Bread crumbs (.5 c)
- Italian seasoning (1 T)
- Chili peppers (2 seeded)
- Basil (6 leaves)
- Egg (1)
- Sun-dried tomatoes (5 chopped)
- Garlic (4 cloves)
- Onion (.5)
- Scallops (6 oz.)
- Coconut oil (4 T)

What to Do

- Coat a pan in 1 T oil and place it on the stove above a burner that has been turned to a high/medium heat.

- Add in the scallops and let them cook until they are completely white.

- In a food processor, mix in 1 T coconut oil, the egg, tomatoes, garlic, and onion before adding in the seasoning, chilies, basil and parsley and process on the medium setting.

- Add in the shrimp, scallops and tuna and process on a low setting.

- Add in the breadcrumbs and keep processing until everything binds together.

- Make the results into patties before adding them to a plate and placing the plate in the refrigerator for at least 2 hours.

- Coat a pan in the remaining oil and place it on the stove above a burner that has been turned to medium heat.

- Cook the patties in the pan until both sides have turned a golden brown.

Cod with Roasted String Beans

Makes enough for: 3

Time required for proper preparation: 10 minutes

Suggested cooking time: 10 minutes

Total required: 20 minutes

What to Use

- Horseradish (as desired)
- Red onion (.5 wedged)
- Black pepper(as desired)
- Red pepper flakes (as desired)
- Dill (3 T chopped)
- Garlic (2 cloves minced)
- Lemon zest (2 T)
- Lemon juice (2 T)
- Extra virgin coconut oil (2 T)
- Codd (16 oz.)

What to Do

- Ensure your oven is heated to 450F.

- Mix the pepper, red pepper flakes, 2 T dill, garlic, lemon zest, lemon juice, and extra virgin coconut oil together in a bowl and combine well. Use half of the results to coat the fish.

- Add the onion and string beans to the remaining oil mixture before spreading the vegetables onto a baking sheet.

- Add the vegetables to the oven and let them cook for 15 minutes before adding the cod to the top of the vegetables face down.

- Let the fish cook for 12 minutes or until the fish looks opaque in its center.

- Season as desired.

Shrimp and Chicken Jambalaya

Makes enough for: 8

Time required for proper preparation: 15 minutes

Suggested cooking time: 6 hours

Total required: 6 hours and 15 minutes

What to Use

- Parsley (2 T)

- Hot sauce (1 T)

- Shrimp (1 lb. peeled, deveined)

- Long grain rice (7 oz.)

- Chicken broth (14 oz. can)

- Tomatoes (14.5 oz. can diced)

- Paprika (.25 tsp)

- Thyme (.5 tsp.)

- Cajun Seasoning (2 tsp.)

- Turkey kielbasa (4 oz. 25-inch slices)

- Garlic (2 cloves minced)

- Celery (1 c chopped)

- Green Bell Pepper (1 c chopped)

- Onion (2 c chopped)

- Chicken thighs (.75 lb. skinless, boneless, 1-inch pieces)

- Chicken breasts (1 lb. skinless, boneless, 1-inch pieces)

- Coconut oil (1 T)

What to Do

- On high heat, preheat a large skillet with a bit of oil. Cook the chicken for about 5 minutes, then place it in the slow cooker.

- Mix the garlic, celery, bell pepper and onion in the skillet before sautéing for 4 minutes. Add the results plus the kielbasa,

- Put this mixture, with Cajun seasoning, thyme, paprika, tomatoes chicken broth, and the turkey kielbasa. Cook on for 6 hours.

- Prepare your rice to your preference, then add the cooked rice and remaining ingredients to the slow cooker. Cook on high for an additional 15 minutes. Garnish with the parsley and enjoy!

Halibut with Mango and Ginger Salsa

Makes enough for: 2

Time required for proper preparation: 15 minutes

Suggested cooking time: 10 minutes

Total required: 25 minutes

What to Use

- Coconut oil (2 T)

- Halibut (1 lb.)

- Mango (1 diced, peeled)

- Red onion (1 chopped)

- Ginger (1 tsp. grated)

- Garlic (2 cloves minced)

- Red pepper (1 chopped)

- Lime (1 juiced)

- Cilantro (.5 bunches)

What to Do

- Season the fish as desired.

- Add the coconut oil to a pan before placing the pan on the stove over a burner set to medium heat.

- Add in the fish and let it cook for approximately 5 minutes on each side.

- Combine the remaining ingredients and add them to the top of the fish, serve hot and enjoy.

Salmon with Roasted Cauliflower

Makes enough for: 2

Time required for proper preparation: 10 minutes

Suggested cooking time: 10 minutes

Total required: 20 minutes

What to Use

- Lemon (.5 wedged)

- Black pepper(as desired)

- Cayenne pepper (1 tsp.)

- Dill (3 T chopped)

- Garlic (2 cloves minced)

- Lemon zest (2 T)

- Lemon juice (2 T)

- Extra virgin coconut oil (2 T)

What to Do

- Ensure your oven is heated to 450F.

- Mix the pepper, red pepper flakes, 2 T dill, garlic, lemon zest, lemon juice, and extra virgin coconut oil together in a bowl and combine well. Use half of the results to coat the fish.

- Add the lemon and cauliflower to the remaining oil mixture before spreading the vegetables onto a baking sheet.

- Add the vegetables to the oven and let them cook for 15 minutes before adding the salmon to the top of the vegetables face down.

- Let the fish cook for 12 minutes or until the fish looks opaque in its center.

- Season as desired.

Crab Salad Cakes

Makes enough for: 4

Time required for proper preparation: 10 minutes

Suggested cooking time: 5 minutes

Total required: 15 minutes

What to Use

- Black pepper (.5 tsp.)

- Salt (.5 tsp.)

- Extra virgin coconut oil (1 T)

- Swiss cheese (.5 c shredded)

- Hot sauce (2 dashes)

- Old Bay seasoning (.25 tsp.)

- Mayonnaise (1 T)

- Lemon juice (4 tsp.)

- Scallion (1 chopped)

- Red bell pepper (.25 c chopped)

- Celery (.3 c chopped)

- Crab meat (8 oz.)

- asparagus spears (4 sliced)

What to Do

- Pace the rack high in the oven and heat your broiler.

- Microwave the asparagus in a covered bowl with 1 tsp. water for 30 seconds.

- Mix in the seasonings as desired as well as the mayonnaise, lemon juice, scallion, bell pepper, celery, and crab.

- For the results into 4 patties and top with the cheese.

- Broil the patties for 3 minutes.

Salmon with Kale

Makes enough for: 4

Time required for proper preparation: 20 minutes

Suggested cooking time: 13 minutes

Total required: 33 minutes

What to Use

- Black pepper (.5 tsp.)

- Salt (.5 tsp.)

- Extra virgin coconut oil (1 T)

- Lemon wedges (4)

- Dill (1 T chopped, fresh)

- Horseradish (2 tsp.)

- Sour cream (.25 c)

- Salmon (1 lb.)

- Kale (1 lb., chopped, stems removed)

- Water (.25 c)

- Chicken broth (1 c)

- Shallot (1 sliced thin)

What to Do

- Add the oil to a pan before placing the pan on the stove over a burner set to medium heat. Mix in.5 lbs. of kale, the water, and the broth before letting the kale wilt for 60 seconds. Mix in the rest of the kale and let it cook for 8 minutes.

- Season the fish as desired before placing it atop the kale, cover the pan and let the fish cook approximately 5 minutes or until done.

- While the fish cooks, in a small bowl, mix together the dill, horseradish and sour cream.

- Top the fish with the results and garnish with the lemon.

Coconut Amino Infused Salmon

Makes enough for: 4

Time required for proper preparation: 10 minutes

Suggested cooking time: 12 minutes

Total required: 22 minutes

What to Use

- Coconut aminos (1.5 c)

- Sesame oil (1 T toasted)

- Coconut oil (1 T)

- Green onions (3 chopped)

- Garlic (3 cloves)

- Salmon filet (4)

- Green beans (.75 lbs.)

- Mushrooms (1 lb.)

- Bell peppers (3 sliced thin, seeds removed)

What to Do

- Ensure your oven has been heated to 450F.

- Add a baking pan to the oven for the salmon as well as two for use with the vegetables.

- Add the garlic, oil, green onions, and coconut aminos to your food processor or blender and go nuts for 30 seconds.

- Coat the salmon using the results.

- In a mixing bowl, and the peppers, mushrooms and green beans and combine thoroughly before adding the remaining sauce and coating well.

- Add the items to their respective pans and let them bake for 12 minutes.

Orange Roughy Fillet

Makes enough for: 2

Time required for proper preparation: 5 minutes

Suggested cooking time: 12 minutes

Total required: 17 minutes

What to Use

- Italian seasoned bread crumbs (2 T)

- Worcestershire sauce (1 tsp.)

- Lemon juice (1.5 tsp.)

- Dijon mustard (1 T)

- Orange roughy (8 oz.)

What to Do

- Start by making sure your oven is heated to 450F.

- Prepare a baking dish (11 x 7) by spraying it with cooking spray before adding in the fish.

- In a small bowl, combine the Worcestershire sauce, lemon juice, and mustard and mix well. Spread the results over the filet evenly before coating in breadcrumbs.

- Place the baking dish in the oven for approximately 12 minutes, you will know the fish is ready when it flakes easily when pressed with a fork.

- Slice in half prior to serving and serve hot.

Baked Shrimp

Makes enough for: 4

Time required for proper preparation: 5 minutes

Suggested cooking time: 10 minutes

Total required: 15 minutes

What to Use

- Shrimp (1 lb. peeled, deveined)

- Low-sodium soy sauce (2 tsp.)

- Olive oil (1 tsp.)

- Creole seasoning (2 tsp.)

- Parsley (2 tsp. dried)

- Honey (1 T)

- Lemon juice (2 T)

What to Do

- Start by making sure your oven is heated to 450F.

- Prepare a baking dish (11 x 7) by spraying it with cooking spray.

- Add in the soy sauce, olive oil, Creole seasoning, dried parsley, and honey and combine thoroughly. Add in the shrimp and toss to coat.

- Place the baking dish in the oven for 8 minutes, stirring every 2 minutes. The shrimp should be a light pink color when ready to serve.

CHAPTER 5

Poultry Recipes

<u>Chicken Cacciatore with Spaghetti Squash</u>

Makes enough for: 6

Time required for proper preparation: 60 minutes

Suggested cooking time: 30 minutes

Total required: 90 minutes

What to Use

- Chicken thighs (4 boneless, skinless, bite-size)

- Onion (1 medium, diced)

- Bell peppers (1 large, bite-size)

- Garlic (2 cloves, minced)

- Dried thyme (.5 tsp)

- Chicken stock (1 cup)

- Diced tomatoes (one 28-ounce can)

- Tomato sauce (one 8-ounce can)

- Dried basil (.5 tsp.)

- Salt (as desired)

- Pepper (as desired)

- Yellow squash (.5, diced)

- Dried oregano (.5 tsp)

- Spaghetti squash (1, small)

What to Do

- Dice the veggies. Set them aside.

- Cut the chicken up. Season it as desired.

- Place the chicken in a Dutch oven and let it brown for about 8 minutes.

- Add in the onion, garlic and bell pepper and let them cook for approximately 5 minutes or until the onions soften.

- Add the chicken tomato sauce, tomatoes, and the chicken stock.

- Season as desired and mix well before letting everything boil.

- Turn the heat to low and let everything cook for 30 minutes.

- Add the yellow squash. Cook between 15 and 30 more minutes.

Celery Fries and Chicken

Makes enough for: 6

Time required for proper preparation: 15 minutes

Suggested cooking time: 20 minutes

Total required: 35 minutes

What to Use - *Chicken*

- Coconut oil (2 T)

- Salt (as needed)

- Chicken breasts (4)

- Pepper (as needed)

What to Use - Celery Fries

- Salt (.5 tsp)

- Pepper (.25 tsp)

- Root celery (1.5 lbs.)

- Coconut oil (2 T)

What to Do

- Ensure your oven is on and turn to 400F.

- Cube the chicken before adding it to a large mixing bowl before adding in 2 T coconut oil and seasoning as needed. Allow the chicken to marinate for at least 15 minutes.

- At the same time, cut the root celery into strips and place it in a large bowl before adding in the remaining coconut oil and seasoning as needed. Shake well to coat.

- Place the celery strips and chicken on a baking sheet before placing the sheet in the oven to bake for 20 minutes.

Chicken Thighs with Turmeric and Cumin

Makes enough for: 2

Time required for proper preparation: 5 minutes

Suggested cooking time: 15 minutes

Total required: 20 minutes

What to Use

- Black pepper (as desired)

- Water (.5 c)

- Hot sauce (1 T)

- Black molasses (1 T)

- Honey (.25 c)

- Coconut oil (2 T)

- Lemon juice (.5 T)

- Turmeric (.5 tsp.)

- Ginger (.5 tsp.)

- Coriander (.5 tsp.)

- Cumin (.5 tsp.)

- Chicken thighs (1 lb.)

What to Do

- Combine the spices in a small bowl and mix well. Use the results to coat the chicken thoroughly before placing it in the Instant Pot cooker pot along with the coconut oil and choose the sauté option, leaving the cooker uncovered. Brown the chicken thighs evenly.

- Remove the chicken from the pot before adding in a little water, be prepared for it to boil quickly. Once the noise dies down, remove the brown bits from the bottom of the Instant Pot cooker pot before returning the chicken to the pot and setting the pressure to high and the time to 15 minutes.

- While the chicken is cooking, combine the lemon, molasses, and honey together in a small bowl.

- Once the timer goes off, select the instant pressure release option and remove the lid.

- Remove the chicken and cover it with foil to keep warm. Turn the Instant Pot cooker back to sauté before adding the honey mixture to the pot and letting everything boil, whisking regularly until the sauce thickens.

- Dip each chicken thigh into the sauce prior to serving.

Chicken Cheese Steak

Makes enough for: 5

Time required for proper preparation: 20 minutes

Suggested cooking time: 5 hours

Total required: 5 hours and 20 minutes

What to Use

- Black pepper (as desired)

- Sea salt (as desired)

- Oopsie Bread (6 slices)

- Steak seasoning (2 T)

- Garlic cloves (2 chopped)

- Provolone cheese (6 slices)

- Green peppers (2 sliced thin)

- Onion (1 sliced)

- Light Coconut oil (2 T)

- Chicken breasts (1 lb.)

What to Do

- Thinly slice the chicken into strips before adding it to a bowl and seasoning with steak seasoning, pepper, and salt as needed.

- Add the coconut oil to the slow cooker before adding in the green peppers as well as the onions and then top it all with the chick.

- Cover the slow cooker and let it cook on low heat for 5 hours.

- Divide the results into 6 servings and add the results to each roll before topping with the cheese and toasting for 2 minutes prior to serving.

Chicken Korma

Makes enough for: 3

Time required for proper preparation: 15 minutes

Suggested cooking time: 30 minutes

Total required: 35 minutes

What to Use

- Chicken breast (16 oz. grilled)

- Cooking cream (100 milliliters 35 percent fat)

- Coconut oil (5 T)

- Cinnamon (1 stick)

- Curry (.5 T)

- Garlic (2 cloves chopped)

- Ginger (2 T grated)

- Cardamom (7 pods)

- Bay (2 leaves)

- Onion (1)

- Cayenne pepper (as desired)

- Coconut oil (30 grams)

- Salt (.5 tsp.)

- Water (3 T)

What to Do

- Cut the onion so that one half is chopped and the other is thinly sliced.

- Place the coconut oil and coconut oil together into a frying pan before adding a medium heat.

- Once the mixture is heated, add in the cardamom pods, bay leaves, and cinnamon sticks and let them sizzle for just a few seconds.

- Add the onion slices into the mixture and allow them to become a light brown.

- Mix the salt, curry, cayenne pepper, garlic, ginger, and chopped onion together well before adding in the cooking cream.

- Add the results to the chicken and mix well.

- Add the water to the pan before letting it simmer for 10 minutes.

Teriyaki Chicken

Makes enough for: 2

Time required for proper preparation: 2 hours and 15 minutes

Suggested cooking time: 25 minutes

Total required: 2 hours and 40 minutes

What to Use

- Black pepper (as needed)

- Salt (as needed)

- Chicken breast (1.5 lbs.)

- Coconut oil (3 T)

- Sweetener (as desired)

- Powdered ginger (1 T)

- Powdered garlic (1 T)

- White vinegar (1 T)

- Worcestershire sauce (1 T)

- Soy sauce (.5 c)

What to Do

- Combine the Worcestershire sauce, coconut oil, sweetener, soy sauce, pepper, salt, ginger, garlic, and vinegar together using a large bowl.

- Add in the chicken, cover the bowl and let the chicken marinate for 2 hours.

- Add the chicken to a frying pan before placing the pan on the stove over a burner turned to a medium heat.

- Cook the chicken until the marinate has nearly completely evaporated and the internal temperature has reached 165 degrees F.

Lemon Chicken

Makes enough for: 3

Time required for proper preparation: 2 hours and 15 minutes

Suggested cooking time: 15 minutes

Total required: 2 hours and 30 minutes

What to Use

- Salt (as desired)

- Pepper (1 tsp.)

- Chicken breast (500 grams)

- Lemon juice (1 T)

- Rosemary (1 T ground)

- Coconut oil (.75 c)

- Olives (15)

- Camembert (50 grams)

What to Do

- Begin by mixing together the pepper, rosemary, coconut oil and lemon juice to make the marinade for the chicken.

- Add the chicken and let it marinate for 2 hours. After it has finished marinating, add salt if you prefer.

- Top the chicken with olives and the camembert prior to serving.

- Place the chicken in a glass baking pan and then place it in the oven for about 15 minutes or until the chicken hits 165F internally.

Zucchini with Feta and Chicken

Makes enough for: 2

Time required for proper preparation: 15 minutes

Suggested cooking time: 20 minutes

Total required: 35 minutes

What to Use

- Salt (as desired)

- Pepper (as desired)

- Chicken breast (500 grams)

- Rosemary (1 T)

- Coconut oil (4 T)

- Lemon Juice (2 T)

- Feta cheese (50 grams)

- Zucchini (2)

What to Do

- Ensure your oven is preheated to 375F

- Prepare the feta cheese, zucchini, and chicken breast by cutting it into cubes.

- Add 1 T of the olive oil into a frying pan and heat it on a high/medium heat before sautéing the zucchini for around 6 minutes.

- Mix together the rest of the oil with the pepper, salt, and rosemary before placing the chicken onto a cooking tray and covering it with the oil mixture.

- Add the feta cheese and zucchini cubes once the chicken has been coated.

- Place tinfoil over the top of the tray, taking special care to leave room in the tinfoil for the steam to escape.

- Bake for 25 minutes.

Off the Cobb Salad

Makes enough for: 1

Time required for proper preparation: 10 minutes

Suggested cooking time: 0 minutes

Total required: 10 minutes

What to Use

- Spinach (1 c)

- Egg (1, hard-boiled)

- Bacon (2 strips)

- Chicken breast (2 oz. grilled)

- Campari tomato (one half of tomato)

- Avocado (one fourth, sliced)

- White vinegar (half of a tsp.)

- Coconut oil (1 T)

What to Do

- Cook the bacon completely and cut or slice into small pieces.

- Chop remaining ingredients into bite-size pieces.

- Place all ingredients, including chicken and bacon, in a bowl, toss ingredients in oil and vinegar.

- Enjoy!

Chicken Casserole

Makes enough for: 4

Time required for proper preparation: 35 minutes

Suggested cooking time: 10 minutes

Total required: 45 minutes

What to Use

- Grass-fed Coconut oil (2 T)

- Salt (as needed)

- Pepper (as needed)

- Heavy whipping cream (1.3 c)

- Separated chicken breast (1.5 lbs.)

- Pitted olives (.5 c)

- Green pesto (4 oz)

- Feta cheese (.5 lbs. shredded)

- Garlic clove (1 chopped)

What to Do

- Ensure your oven is on and turned to 400F.

- Mix together the pesto and the heavy cream in a mixing bowl.

- Add the cheese, chicken, olives, and garlic to a baking dish and cover with the peso/cream mixture.

- Add the dish to the oven and let it cook 30 minutes.

BLT Chicken Salad

Makes enough for: 1

Time required for proper preparation: 15 minutes

Suggested cooking time: 0 minutes

Total required: 15 minutes

What to Use

- Boneless chicken breast (1, grilled)

- Leaf lettuce (2 c, chopped)

- Tomato (.5 small)

- Swiss cheese (.5-oz., julienned)

- Bacon (1-2 strips, crisp and crumbled)

- Egg (.5 hard-boiled, sliced in half)

- Ranch dressing (2 T)

- Black pepper (dash)

- Parsley (pinch, fresh, chopped, optional)

- Sliced cucumber (chopped, optional)

- Chives (chopped, optional)

- Green peppers (slivered, optional)

- Avocado (chopped, optional)

- Sunflower seeds (optional)

What to Do

- Add the sliced chicken to a large plate covered in lettuce.

- Top the chicken with the remaining ingredients.

California Grilled Chicken
Avocado-Mango Salad

Makes enough for: 4

Time required for proper preparation: 15 minutes

Suggested cooking time: 0 minutes

Total required: 15 minutes

What to Use

- Chicken breast (12-oz. breast, grilled, sliced)

- Avocado (1 c, diced)

- Mango (1 c, diced from 1.5 mangos)

- Red onion (2 T)

- Red Coconut oil lettuce (6 c)

What to Use - Vinaigrette

- Balsamic vinegar (2 T white)

- Salt (as desired)

- Pepper (as desired)

- Coconut oil (2 T)

What to Do

- Whisk all vinaigrette ingredients together. Set aside.

- Fill 4 salad plates with baby greens.

- Toss the onion, mango, avocado, and chicken together.

- Plate the chicken atop the baby greens and top with vinaigrette prior to serving.

Chicken Curry

Makes enough for: 6

Time required for proper preparation: 30 minutes

Suggested cooking time: 40 minutes

Total required: 70 minutes

What to Use

- Chicken breasts (1.5 breasts)

- Cauliflower (1 head)

- Onion powder (.5 tsp.)

- Thai Kitchen Lite Coconut Milk (1 can)

- Hot curry powder (2 T)

- Garam masala (1 T)

- Coconut oil (.5 T)

- Green beans (2 c, frozen)

- Garlic powder (.5 tsp)

- Salt (as desired)

- Pepper (as desired)

What to Do

- Cut up the chicken into chunks.

- Coat the chicken chunks in half curry powder and half garam masala.

- Take the chicken out and put it into a deep pot. Leave the burned pieces and coconut oil in the frying pan because they are flavorful.

- Add coconut milk to the frying pan and scratch off all of the burned bits.

- Pour the coconut milk and the burned bits over the chicken that is in the deep pot.

- Add the remaining spices.

- Boil on a low/medium heat for half an hour.

- Add green beans. Continue cooking, uncovered to let the sauce thicken.

- Meanwhile, boil the cauliflower in water and 1 T of coconut oil in a separate pot.

- Mash the cauliflower until it is in small pieces. Season as needed.

Spaghetti Squash Chicken Alfredo

Makes enough for: 4

Time required for proper preparation: 15 minutes

Suggested cooking time: 20 minutes

Total required: 35 minutes

What to Use - Meal

- Garlic powder (1 tsp.)

- Sea salt (.5 tsp.)

- Basil for garnish

- Medium spaghetti squash (1)

- Chicken breast(1 lb.)

- Coconut oil (2 T)

- Juice of half a lemon

What to Use - Sauce

- Bone broth (.25 c)

- Medium cauliflower chopped (1)

- Coconut milk (.25 c)

- Coconut oil (1 T)

- Garlic powder (1 tsp.)

- Sea salt (.5 tsp.)

What to Do

- Preheat the oven to 400F

- Slice the squash in half and spoon out the seeds. Bake in the oven for 45- 50 minutes or until the strands easily pull.

- Season the chicken breast with lemon, salt, and garlic and allow to marinate for about an hour in the fridge.

- Heat cooking fat of choice over medium heat and add the chicken.

- Add the cauliflower to a medium pot and fill about 60 percent of the way with water.

- Heat the cauliflower on medium heat and bring to a low simmer for about 8-10 minutes or until cauliflower is soft.

- Strain the cauliflower and allow it to cool.

- Add the cooled cauliflower to a high-speed blender with the remainder of the ingredients and blend until smooth.

- Either scoop the squash out of the shell or keep it in.

- Add the sauce and combine, reserving some to add over the top.

- Add the sliced chicken, some extra sauce, and basil for garnish.

- Serve and enjoy!

Low-Carb Pizza

Makes enough for: 2

Time required for proper preparation: 15 minutes

Suggested cooking time: 30 minutes

Total required: 45 minutes

What to Use

- Salt (.5 tsp.)

- Egg (1 large)

- White wine vinegar (1 tsp.)

- Cream cheese (2 T)

- Almond flour (.75 c)

- Mozzarella cheese (2 c divided, shredded)

- Grilled chicken (.5 lb.)

- Coconut oil (1 T grass fed)

- Oregano (.5 tsp. dried)

- Tomato sauce (.5 c unsweetened)

What to Do

- Start by making sure your oven is heated to 400F.

- Add the cream cheese and mozzarella cheese to a small pan before placing this pan on the stove on top of a burner set to medium heat.

- Stir to mix and continue stirring until both kinds of cheese have melted. Add in the .5 tsp. salt, the egg, and 1 tsp. white wine vinegar and mix thoroughly.

- Coat your hands in oil before taking the dough and flattening it out onto parchment paper so that it ends up being roughly 8 inches round. A rolling pin will also work if available.

- Using a fork, create a number of holes in the dough to prevent it from rising before placing it on a baking sheet and letting it bake approximately 11 minutes.

- Add the toppings to the pizza, starting with the sauce, before placing it on a baking sheet and baking for 15 minutes.

- Top with oregano prior to serving.

CHAPTER 6

Beef Recipes

Fajita and Poblano Kabobs

Makes enough for: 3

Time required for proper preparation: 60 minutes

Suggested cooking time: 20 minutes

Total required: 80 minutes

What to Use - Marinade

- Black pepper (as needed)

- Salt (as needed)

- Flank steak (1 lb. sliced thin)

- Red pepper flakes (.25 tsp.)

- Sweet paprika (.25 tsp.)

- Oregano (.25 tsp.)

- Garlic powder (.25 tsp.)

- Lime juice (.5 T)

- Coconut aminos (.25 cups)

What to Use - Kabobs

- Red onion (.5 chopped)

- Red bell pepper (1 chopped)

- Yellow bell pepper (1 chopped)

What to Use - Poblano Pesto

- Coconut oil (2 T)

- Lime juice (.5 T)

- Cilantro (.5 cups)

- Poblano pepper (1 roasted)

What to Do

- Place the marinade ingredients as well as the steak into a dish with a lid and ensure the meat is well coated. Let the marinade chill for at least 2 hours.

- Skewer the meat and vegetables as desired before heating a grill pan in the oil and place it on the stove above a burner that has been turned to medium heat. Brush each kabob with the marinade before cooking each side for approximately 4 minutes.

- As the kabobs are cooking, add the pesto ingredients to a blender and blend well.

- Add the pesto to the kabobs prior to serving.

Steak Salad

Makes enough for: 4

Time required for proper preparation: 15 minutes

Suggested cooking time: 0 minutes

Total required: 15 minutes

What to Use

- Pepper (as desired)
- Salt (as desired)
- Carrots (3 sliced)
- Red leaf lettuce (1 head torn)
- Dijon mustard (1 T)
- Coconut oil (2 T)
- Radishes (8 quartered)
- Garlic (1 clove minced)
- White wine vinegar (2 T)
- Snap peas (8 oz. halved, steamed)
- Skirt steak (1 lb. halved)

What to Do

- Heat your broiler before placing the steak on top of a baking sheet lined with tinfoil (seasoned as desired) and broiling the steak for 4 minutes. Remove the steak from the broil and tent it in the tinfoil to keep it warm.

- Combine the garlic, mustard, vinegar, and oil and whisk well to combine thoroughly. Toss the lettuce using half the dressing.

- Slice the steak and place it and the remaining ingredients on top of the tossed salad. Top with dressing prior to serving.

Orange Beef Stew

Makes enough for: 4

Time required for proper preparation: 15 minutes

Suggested cooking time: 8 hours

Total required: 8 hours and 15 minutes

What to Use

- Salt (as needed)

- Pepper (as needed)

- Rutabagas (3 spiralized)

- Sage (1 T chopped fine)

- Thyme (1 T chopped fine)

- Rosemary (1 T chopped fine)

- Bay leaves (2)

- Cinnamon (2 tsp. ground)

- Water (4 c)

- Balsamic vinegar (.25 c)

- Orange juice (.5 c)

- Orange zest (1 orange)

- Garlic (2 cloves minced)

- Celery (1 stalked diced)

- Carrot (1 diced)

- Onion (1 diced)

- Coconut oil (3 T)

- Beef stew meat (900 g cubed)

What to Do

- Add everything except for the sage, thyme, rutabagas, and rosemary to the slow cooker. Adjust the slow cooker temperature to low and leave it be, covered, for 8 hours.

- About 10 minutes prior to serving remove the bay leaves and add in the remaining ingredients.

Beef and Shirataki Noodles

Makes enough for: 2

Time required for proper preparation: 10 minutes

Suggested cooking time: 10 minutes

Total required: 20 minutes

What to Use

- Black pepper (as desired)

- Yellow onion (.5)

- Mozzarella cheese (2 oz. shredded)

- Shirataki noodles (.5 c)

- Ground beef (.75 lbs.)

- Coconut oil (2 T)

- Water (.5 c)

What to Do

- Turn the Instant Pot cooker to sauté before adding in the coconut oil. Once it is heated, add in the onion and allow it to cook approximately 5 minutes until it is brown and soft. Add in the beef and brown it as well.

- Add in the water and the shirataki noodles before turning the Instant Pot cooker to steam and letting the shirataki noodles cook approximately 5 minutes or until done.

- Once the timer goes off, and in the cheese and let it melt slightly prior to serving.

Shepherd's Pie

Makes enough for: 12

Time required for proper preparation: 15 minutes

Suggested cooking time: 30 minutes

Total required: 45 minutes

What to Use

- Water (1 c)

- Coconut oil (4 T)

- Cauliflower (1 head)

- Cream cheese (4 oz.)

- Mozzarella (1 c)

- Egg (1)

- Salt (as desired)

- Pepper (as desired)

- Garlic powder (1 T)

- Ground beef (2 lbs.)

- Peas (1 c)

- Carrots (1 c)

- Mushrooms (8 oz. sliced)

- Beef broth (1 c)

What to Do

- Pour the water into the Instant Pot and arrange the cauliflower on top with the leaves and stems removed. Close the lid and set approximately 5 minutes or until done using high pressure.

- Quick release and add the cauliflower to a blender. Add the cream cheese, Coconut oil, mozzarella, egg, pepper, and salt. Blend until smooth.

- Drain the water from the Instant Pot. Toss in the beef, carrots, peas, garlic powder, and broth with a bit more pepper and salt to your liking.

- Blend in the cauliflower mixture and cook ten minutes on high (manual function).

- Serve and enjoy!

Cabbage Roll 'Unstuffed' Soup

Makes enough for: 9

Time required for proper preparation: 10 minutes

Suggested cooking time: 30 minutes

Total required: 40 minutes

What to Use

- Garlic (2 cloves minced)

- Onion (1 diced)

- Ground beef (1.5 lb.)

- Bragg"s Aminos (.25 c)

- Tomato sauce (8 oz.)

- Beef broth (3 c.)

- Worcestershire sauce „keto" approved/another substitute (3 t.)

- Diced tomatoes (14 oz.)

- Chopped cabbage (1)

- Parsley (.5 t)

- Pepper (as desired)

- Salt (as desired)

What to Do

- Add everything to the pressure cooker and mix well.

- Program the unit on the soup function. Natural release the soup for about ten minutes, and quick release the rest of the steam. Stir and serve.

Greek Meatballs with Tomato Sauce

Makes enough for: 6

Time required for proper preparation: 35 minutes

Suggested cooking time: 15 minutes

Total required: 50 minutes

What to Use - Meatballs

- Egg (1 slightly beaten)

- Ground beef (1 lb.)

- Chopped parsley (.25 c.)

- Finely chopped onion (.5 c.)

- Arborio rice (.3 c.)

- Salt (as desired)

- Pepper (as desired)

What to Use - Sauce

- Water (1 c)

- Tomatoes (14 oz. diced)

- Smoked paprika (.5 t)

- Cinnamon (.5 t)

- Dried oregano (1 t)

- Cloves (.25 t ground)

- Salt (as desired)

- Pepper (as desired)

What to Do

- Mix all of the meatballs fixings, shaping into eight to ten balls. Arrange in a single layer in the pot.

- Mix the sauce components in a dish and pour over the prepared meatballs.

- Program the Instant Pot for 15 minutes under high-pressure and release the pressure with the natural release option.

- Remove the meatballs and blend the sauce until smooth with an immersion blender. Pour over the meatballs, garnish, and serve.

Bunless Burger

Makes enough for: 6

Time required for proper preparation: 35 minutes

Suggested cooking time: 15 minutes

Total required: 50 minutes

What to Use

- Grass-fed Ground Beef (1.5 lbs.)

- Pepper (as desired)

- Pepper Jack Cheese (4 thick slices)

- Bacon (8 slices)

- Large Red Onion, Sliced (1 total)

- Romaine Lettuce Leaves (8 total)

- Salt (as desired)

What to Do

- Warm ground beef to room temperature, and then shape beef into 4 patties. Use thumb to make an indent in the center of each patty so they cook evenly.

- Take a broiler pan and place each patty, thumbprint side facing up. Season as desired and heat oven''s broiler to high.

Once hot, place patties on the center rack and broil for 7 minutes.

- When done, the patties should be golden brown and cooked. Remove from oven and top with a slice of pepper jack cheese on each. Replace in oven and broil to thoroughly, taking care to watch for signs of doneness so they don"t burn.

- Add the bacon to the skillet before placing the skillet on top of a burner set to medium heat and let it cook as needed.

Stir Fry with Cabbage

Makes enough for: 4

Time required for proper preparation: 20 minutes

Suggested cooking time: 25 minutes

Total required: 45 minutes

What to Use

- Wasabi paste (.5 T)

- Keto mayonnaise (1 c)

- Sesame oil (1 T)

- Ginger (1 T grated)

- Chili flakes (1 tsp.)

- Scallions (3 sliced)

- Garlic (2 cloves)

- White wine vinegar (1 T)

- Black pepper (.25 tsp. ground)

- Onion powder (1 tsp.)

- Salt (1 tsp.)

- Beef (1.3 lbs. ground)

- Coconut oil (5 oz. grass fed)

- Cabbage (1.6 lbs. shredded)

What to Do

- Add 3 oz. coconut oil to a frying pan before placing the pan on a burner set to a high/medium heat.

- Add the cabbage to the frying pan and let it cook, taking care to prevent it from browning. Season using vinegar and spices before continuing to stir and fry an additional 2 minutes before removing the cabbage from heat.

- Add the remainder of the coconut oil to the frying pan before adding in the ginger, chili flakes, and garlic and sautéing for 3 minutes.

- Add in the meat and season using pepper, salt, and sesame oil and ensure everything is hot prior to serving.

- Combine the wasabi paste and the mayo and add the results to the stir fry prior to serving.

Ground Beef, Veggies, and Noodles

Makes enough for: 6

Time required for proper preparation: 10 minutes

Suggested cooking time: 10 minutes

Total required: 20 minutes

What to Use

- Oil (1 T)

- Ground beef (1 lb.)

- Bell peppers (1 c chopped)

- Garlic (2 cloves)

- Onion (.5 c chopped)

- Baby spinach (4 c)

- Shirataki noodles (2 packages)

- Parmesan cheese (.5 c grated)

What to Do

- Prepare the Instant Pot on the sauté function and add the oil when hot.

- Add the garlic, ground beef, onions, peppers, and spinach. Scrape the browning bits from the bottom and secure the lid.

- Use the high-pressure setting for three minutes and quick-release the pressure. Empty the sauce over the noodles and garnish with the cheese.

Chili

Makes enough for: 6

Time required for proper preparation: 25 minutes

Suggested cooking time: 3 hours

Total required: 3 hours and 25 minutes

What to Use

- Worcestershire sauce (1 tsp.)

- Cayenne pepper (.5 tsp.)

- Oregano (1 tsp.)

- Paprika (2 tsp.)

- Garlic (2 tsp. minced)

- Fish sauce (2 tsp.)

- Cumin (1.5 tsp.)

- Chili powder (2 T + 1 tsp.)

- Coconut oil (2 T)

- Soy sauce (2 T)

- Tomato paste (.3 c)

- Beef broth (1 c)

- Green pepper (1 chopped)

- Onion (1 chopped)

- Ground beef (2 lbs.)

What to Do

- In a small bowl, combine the Worcestershire sauce, cayenne pepper, oregano, paprika, cumin, fish sauce, 2 T chili powder, and soy sauce and mix well to form a sauce.

- Add the garlic, green pepper and onion to a skillet before placing it on the stove over a burner turned to medium heat and letting them sauté until you can begin to see through the onions.

- Add everything to a slow cooker and combine thoroughly.

- Cover the slow cooker and let it cook on high heat for 2.5 hours and then uncovered for an additional 30 minutes.

Quarter Pound Burger

Makes enough for: 2

Time required for proper preparation: 10 minutes

Suggested cooking time: 8 minutes

Total required: 18 minutes

What to Use

- Basil (half a tsp.)

- Cayenne (fourth a tsp.)

- Crushed red pepper (half a tsp.)

- Salt (half a tsp.)

- Lettuce (2 large leaves)

- Coconut oil (2 T)

- Egg (1 large)

- Sriracha (1 T)

- Onion (fourth of whole onion)

- Plum tomato (half of a whole tomato)

- Mayo (1 T)

- Pickled jalapenos (1 T, sliced)

- Bacon (1 strip)

- Ground beef (.5 lbs.)

- Bacon (1 strip)

What to Do

- Knead mean for about three minutes.

- Chop bacon, jalapeno, tomato, and onion into fine pieces. (shown below)

- Knead in mayo, sriracha, egg, and chopped ingredients, and spices into the meat.

- Separate meat into four even pieces and flatten them (not thinly, just press on the tops to create a flat surface). Place a T of Coconut oil on top of two of the meat pieces. Take the pieces that do not have Coconut oil of them and set them on top of the coconut oiled ones (basically creating a Coconut oil and meat sandwich). Seal the sides together, concealing the coconut oil within.

- Throw the patties on the grill (or in a pan) for about 5 minutes on each side. Caramelize some onions if you want too!

- Prepare large leaves of lettuce by spreading some mayo onto them. Once patties are finished, place them on one half of the lettuce, add your desired burger toppings, and fold the other half over of the lettuce leaf over the patty.

- Burger time!

Brussel Sprouts and Hamburger

Makes enough for: 3

Time required for proper preparation: 30 minutes

Suggested cooking time: 15 minutes

Total required: 45 minutes

What to Use

- Black pepper (as desired)

- Sea salt (as desired)

- Italian seasoning (1 T)

- Shredded cheese (5.3 oz.)

- Coconut oil (2 oz.)

- Sour cream (4 T)

- Brussel sprouts (1 lb. halved)

- Bacon (oz. diced)

- Ground beef (1 lb.)

What to Do

- Ensure your oven is heated to 425F.

- Add the Brussel sprouts and bacon to a frying pan and place the pan on the stove over a burner turned to high/medium. Season before adding in the sour cream and add the results to the baking dish.

- Add in the ground beef, herbs, and cheese.

- Add the baking sheet to oven and let it cook for 15 minutes.

Beef Casserole

Makes enough for: 4

Time required for proper preparation: 20 minutes

Suggested cooking time: 25 minutes

Total required: 45 minutes

What to Use

- Black pepper (as desired)
- Sea salt (as desired)
- Guacamole (1 c)
- Coconut oil (2 oz.)
- Scallion (1 chopped fine)
- Crème Fraiche (1 c)
- Cheese (7 oz. shredded)
- Jalapenos (2 oz.)
- Tomatoes (7 oz. crushed)
- Ground beef (1.5 lbs.)
- Cayenne pepper (1 pinch)
- Onion powder (1 tsp.)

- Garlic powder (1 tsp.)

- Cumin (1 tsp. ground)

- Paprika powder (2 tsp.)

- Chili powder (2 tsp.)

What to Do

- Ensure your oven is heated to 400F.

- Add the beef and tomatoes to a pan before placing it on the stove over a burner turned to a high/medium heat and then top with all the seasonings and mix well.

- Add the results to the baking dish before topping with the cheese and jalapenos. Place the dish on the top rack of the oven and let it bake approximately 20 minutes.

- Top with sour cream and chives and serve with guacamole.

Low-Carb Meatballs

Makes enough for: 2

Time required for proper preparation: 15 minutes

Suggested cooking time: 8 minutes

Total required: 23 minutes

What to Use

- Black pepper (as desired)

- Mozzarella cheese (.25 c)

- Garlic (1 T minced)

- Parmesan cheese (.25 c grated)

- Ground beef (.5 lbs.)

- Coconut oil (4 T)

What to Do

- Combine everything together in a large bowl before forming the results into 4 meatballs (2 per serving).

- Turn the Instant Pot cooker to sauté before adding in the oil and allowing it to warm up fully.

- Cook each meatball for approximately 2 minutes per side.

Instant Pot Steak

Makes enough for: 2

Time required for proper preparation: 15 minutes

Suggested cooking time: 35 minutes

Total required: 50 minutes

What to Use

- Worcestershire sauce (1.5 tsp)

- Flank steak (1 lb.)

- ACV (2 T)

- Coconut oil (.25 c)

- Onion soup mix (1 T)

What to Do

- Set to sauté.

- Brown the steak on both sides.

- Add onion soup mix, coconut oil, Worcestershire, and vinegar.

- Lock and seal lid.

- Set to meat/stew for 35 minutes. Carefully release pressure.

Maple Brisket

Makes enough for: 2

Time required for proper preparation: 15 minutes

Suggested cooking time: 40 minutes

Total required: 55 minutes

What to Use

- Beef brisket (1 lb.)

- Maple sugar (1 T)

- Pepper (as desired)

- Onion powder (.5 tsp.)

- Paprika (.25 tsp.)

- Mustard powder (.5 tsp.)

- Beef broth (1 c)

- Liquid smoke (1.5 tsp.)

- Thyme sprigs (2)

What to Do

- Mix dry spices together and coat brisket.

- Set pot to sauté. Grease with oil and brown brisket. Lay brisket fat side up, and add thyme, broth, and liquid smoke.

- Cook on high for 40 minutes. Once finished, let pressure release naturally. Remove and cover with foil.

- Optional: Turn to sauté and reduce leftover liquid.

- Slice brisket and drizzle with liquid.

Rosemary Veal

Makes enough for: 2

Time required for proper preparation: 15 minutes

Suggested cooking time: 5 hours

Total required: 5 hours and 15 minutes

What to Use

- Leg of lamb (1)

- Rosemary (2 sticks fresh)

- Pumpkin (1 medium quartered)

- Potatoes (2 c chopped)

- Carrots (2 sliced)

- Celery (1 stock sliced)

- Shallot (1 sliced)

- Vegetable broth (.75 c)

- Garlic (2 cloves sliced)

- Rosemary (.25 tsp dried)

- Coconut oil (.5 tsp)

- Whole wheat flour (2 tsp)

- Dijon mustard (1 tsp)

- Salt (as desired)

- Pepper (as desired)

What to Do

- You can cook this recipe either in the inside of your oven or in a slow cooker. If you decide to cook in an oven, you should increase the stock you use by up to 1 or 1.5 c and then also reduce the cooking time between either 1.5 hours or 2 hours than what you would in a slow cooker. For oven cooking, cook at 285F.

- To get started with your seasoned oil, cook on low heat in a frying pan so that the garlic and the shallot start to sizzle but do not turn brown. Next, remove the garlic and shallot and throw them away. Keep the remaining oil in the pan.

- Add in the vegetables in order to sauté them. Cook the vegetables until they start to appear brown over medium heat. You will then remove the vegetables and then place them inside the slow cooker if you choose to use one for this recipe.

- Next, remove any fat pieces from the lamb and then cut small slits in the meat. Use salt and pepper in order to season the meat and then insert the sprigs of rosemary.

- Brown the lamb in your seasoned oil. You will then place the veal on top of the prepared vegetables that are resting inside the slow cooker. You should save a stick of rosemary and then break it in two pieces to place on both sides of the lamb.

- Mix together the flour and the mustard together and then add it into the stock with the vegetables and veal. You will want to stir the mixture together until it becomes thick.

- Depending on the size of your veal, you should set your slow cooker between 4 or 5 hours to cook.

Beef Tenderloin with Couscous

Makes enough for: 2

Time required for proper preparation: 30 minutes

Suggested cooking time: 2 hours and 30 minutes

Total required: 3 hours

What to Use - Beef

- Beef tenderloin (2 fillets)
- Coconut oil (2 T)
- Pepper (as desired)
- Salt (as desired)

What to Use - Couscous

- Whole wheat couscous (1 c)
- Cherry tomatoes (2 halved)
- Shallot (1)
- Coconut oil (1 T)
- Lemon juice (2 tsp.)
- Cumin (1 tsp. ground)
- Chickpeas (14 oz.)

- Parsley (2 T freshly chopped)

- Salt (as desired)

- Pepper (as desired)

What to Do

- Drain and rinse the chickpeas.

- Set the Sous Vide Supreme to 130F (med-rare).

- Sprinkle the steaks with the pepper and salt. Seal each one in its own bag.

- Add them to the bath – not touching.

- Cover for 2 to 2.5 hours. When done, transfer them to a pan coated in the oil. Let them rest a few minutes before slicing.

- Make the couscous and combine with the chickpeas, tomatoes, coconut oil, lemon juice, and parsley. Sprinkle with the pepper and salt.

- Spoon the couscous onto a plate or bowl and top with the beef.

- Garnish with parsley and lemon slices.

Beef Tenderloin with Pesto and Asparagus

Makes enough for: 4

Time required for proper preparation: 20 minutes

Suggested cooking time: 20 minutes

Total required: 40 minutes

What to Use

- Beef tenderloin (4, 6 oz. pieces)

- Kosher salt – divided (1 T)

- Black pepper (as desired)

- Coconut oil (.25 c.)

- Garlic cloves (5 large)

- Parmesan cheese (2 T grated)

- Lemon (1 zest and juice)

- Asparagus spears (16-20)

- Basil leaves (1 c. fresh)

What to Do

- Set the temperature in the water bath to 135F.

- Sprinkle the meat with pepper and salt and place into two pouches. Vacuum seal. Set the timer for two hours.

- In boiling water on the stovetop, blanch the basil for 30 seconds. Transfer it to an ice bath. Drain and chop. Do the same for the garlic (30 seconds, and dip).

- Combine the basil, garlic, parmesan cheese, and one tsp of salt, along with the oil in a blender until smooth.

- Add the juice and adjust to your liking.

- Add the asparagus to a cooking bag in a single layer. Season with salt if desired and add a bit of the pesto. Vacuum seal and cook beside the meat for 15 minutes.

- Remove the packs and sear the meat for 30-45 seconds per side on a well- greased grill.

- Enjoy with the asparagus and more pesto.

CHAPTER 7

Vegan Recipes

<u>Zoodles</u>

Several of the recipes in this chapter center around zoodles. Zoodles are simply zucchini in the shape of noodles. They will allow you to enjoy all of your favorite pasta recipes without the carbs. These "noodles" are low in calories and carbs, yet they will taste just as delicious as any other noodle you could try. Plus, they can be made very quickly, ready to serve in minutes, or as a part of meal prep. You will want to ensure that the sauces you choose to use have high amounts of fat and protein to make up most of the energy from this meal, as zucchini alone is not high in either.

Makes enough for: 2

Time required for proper preparation: 5 minutes Suggested cooking time: 0 minutes

Total required: 5 minutes

What to Use

- Zucchini (4 organic)

What to Do - Zoodle Creation

- If you have access to a spiralizer, use it to create noodles of zucchini. If you do not own a spiralizer, this recipe is still very simple. Just slice the zucchini into long thin strips. You may also wish to use a cheese and vegetable grater to get the desired noodle effect.

- Serve the zoodles as they are or let them boil for two minutes in a pan of water to warm them up and soften them a bit. Alternately, you may wish to sauté them in a bit of coconut oil or Coconut oil for a minute or two to give them a little crispness.

- Serve the zoodles in place of the traditional noodles in your favorite pasta dishes.

Biryani

Makes enough for: 6

Time required for proper preparation: 15 minutes

Suggested cooking time: 15 minutes

Total required: 30 minutes

What to Use

- Black pepper (as desired)
- Sea salt (as desired)
- Garam masala (.5 tsp)
- Coconut oil (1 tsp)
- Shelled peas (1 c)
- Water (2.5 c)
- Coriander (.5 tsp ground)
- Chili powder (1 tsp)
- Turmeric (1.5 tsp)
- Carrots (2 quartered)
- Potatoes (2 quartered)
- Bay leaves (2 torn)

- Cumin seeds (.5 tsp)

- Onion (1 sliced thin)

- Vegetable oil (3 T)

- White rice long grain (2 c)

What to Do

- Add the rice to a large pot and cover it with three to four inches of water before allowing it to soak for about 20 minutes. Drain and set aside.

- Add the oil to your pressure cooker and set it over medium heat. Add in the onion, bay leaves, and cumin seeds and let everything cook about 5 minutes until the onion is nearly see through.

- Mix in the carrots and potatoes and let them cook an additional 5 minutes and the potatoes have begun to brown. Add in the coriander, turmeric and chili powder and let everything cook 1 additional minute.

- Add the rice to the pressure cooker and ensure it is well covered in the boil before adding in the peas and water. Mix in the garam masala, oil, and salt before sealing the cooker and turning it to high pressure. Let everything cook for 5 minutes before removing from heat.

- Allow the pressure to naturally release and fluff the rice with a fork prior to serving.

Greek Mixed Roasted Vegetables

Makes enough for: 4

Time required for proper preparation: 15 minutes

Suggested cooking time: 45 minutes

Total required: 60 minutes

What to Use - Vegetables

- 1 eggplant (peeled and diced .75-inch

- Black pepper(as desired)

- Kosher sea salt (as desired)

- Extra virgin olive oil (2 T)

- Garlic (2 cloves minced)

- Onion (1 peeled, diced 1-inch)

- Bell pepper (2 red, yellow, diced, 1-inch)

What to Use - Dressing

- Coconut oil (.25 c)

- Lemon juice (.3 c squeezed fresh)

- Black pepper (as desired)

- Kosher sea salt (as desired)

- Basil (15 leaves)

- Scallions (4 minced)

What to Do

- Ensure your oven is heated to 425F.

- One a sheet pan, combine the garlic, onion, yellow bell pepper, red bell pepper, and eggplant before seasoning using the pepper, salt, and coconut oil.

- Add the pan to the oven and let it cook for 40 minutes, using a spatula to flip everything after 20 minutes.

- As the vegetables are cooking, combine the pepper, salt, coconut oil, and lemon juice together in a small bowl, add the results to the vegetables as soon as they are ready.

- Let the pan cool completely before adding in the basil, feta, and scallions. Season prior to serving.

Autumn Roasted Green Beans

Makes enough for: 4

Time required for proper preparation: 15 minutes

Suggested cooking time: 30 minutes

Total required: 45 minutes

What to Use

- Walnuts (.5 c toasted)

- Cranberries (.5 c dried)

- Black pepper (as desired)

- Kosher sea salt (as desired)

- Lemon juice (2 tsp.)

- Lemon zest (1 tsp.)

- Sugar (.25 tsp.)

- Coconut oil (2 T)

- Garlic (4 cloves, quartered and peeled)

- Green beans (2 lbs. stems trimmed)

What to Do

- Preheat your oven to 350F and crack and smash the walnuts into chunks.

- Spread the walnuts onto a baking sheet and toast them for 10 minutes.

- Increase the temperature on the oven to 450F.

- Cover a baking sheet with a rim using aluminum foil.

- In a mixing bowl, combine the sugar, pepper, salt and coconut oil before coating the garlic and green beans thoroughly.

- Place the beans onto a baking sheet and spread them out to ensure they cook well. Place the sheet into the oven and let the beans bake for 15 minutes, before stirring with a spatula and roasting another 10 minutes.

- Mix in the lemon juice, pepper and salt prior to serving.

Roasted Summer Squash

Makes enough for: 4

Time required for proper preparation: 5 minutes

Suggested cooking time: 30 minutes

Total required: 35 minutes

What to Use

- Zucchini (3)

- Yellow squash (3)

- Kosher salt (1.5 T)

- Black pepper (.5 T)

- Coconut oil (2 T)

What to Do

- Ensure your oven is heated to 400F

- Peel vegetables and cut into.25 inch thick slices.

- Assemble vegetables on a baking sheet or pan and drizzle coconut oil on top. Sprinkle with seasoning as desired

- Bake at 400F for 30 minutes.

Savory Baked Acorn Squash

Makes enough for: 4

Time required for proper preparation: 5 minutes

Suggested cooking time: 30 minutes

Total required: 35 minutes

What to Use

- Acorn squash (1)

- Kosher salt (as desired)

- Black pepper (as desired)

- Coconut oil (2 tsp.)

- Smoked paprika (as desired)

What to Do

- Ensure your oven is heated to 425F.

- Cut acorn squash in half lengthwise, then cut halves into quarters lengthwise. Scoop out seeds and discard.

- Place the squash on baking sheet and drizzle coconut oil over the top of each quarter. Scatter with the smoked paprika, salt, and pepper and bake in the oven for 30 minutes.

Roasted Brussels Sprouts

Makes enough for: 4

Time required for proper preparation: 5 minutes

Suggested cooking time: 15 minutes

Total required: 20 minutes

What to Use

- Sea salt (.25 tsp.)

- Black pepper (.25 tsp.)

- Brussel sprouts (.75lbs. sliced in half length-wise)

- Coconut oil (1.5 T.)

What to Do

- Ensure your oven is heated to 400F. Cut Brussels sprouts in half and place in a medium-sized bowl. Drizzle the coconut oil over the Brussels sprouts and then toss with the sea salt and black pepper until evenly coated.

- Pour Brussels sprouts onto a baking sheet and make sure they are evenly spaced so that they will roast easily.

- Place the sheet in the oven and let it cook approximately 10 minutes before stirring well and returning it to the oven for 10 minutes more. Season as desired They will keep in the fridge for 3-4 days, or in the freezer for 2-3 months.

Roasted Rosemary Potatoes

Makes enough for: 6

Time required for proper preparation: 10 minutes

Suggested cooking time: 25 minutes

Total required: 35 minutes

What to Use

- Garlic (1 head)
- Rosemary (3 sprigs)
- Thyme (3 sprigs)
- Baby potatoes (20 oz.)
- Parsley (2 T chopped)
- Sea salt (as desired)
- Black pepper (as desired)
- Coconut oil (2 T)

What to Do

- Ensure your oven is heated to 450F.
- Separate garlic cloves and remove the papery skin holding them together, but do not peel.

- Add the rosemary, thyme, baby potatoes, parsley, garlic, and coconut oil together in a large bowl, coating well.

- Add the results to a jelly roll pan that has been lined with tinfoil before topping with pepper and salt. Place the pan in the oven and let the potatoes bake approximately 25 minutes, stirring at the 12-minute mark.

- Season with additional pepper and salt prior to serving.

Sweet Potato Wedges

Makes enough for: 6

Time required for proper preparation: 10 minutes

Suggested cooking time: 30 minutes

Total required: 40 minutes

What to Use

- Salt (1 tsp.)

- Cracked black pepper (1 tsp.)

- Garlic powder (.5 tsp.)

- Sweet potatoes (4 medium, peeled, each cut into 6 wedges

- Rosemary (1 T chopped, fresh)

- Coconut oil (2 T)

What to Do

- Preheat oven to 450F.

- In a mixing bowl, combine the coconut oil, rosemary, sweet potatoes, garlic powder, black pepper, and salt together and ensure the potatoes are coated well.

- Add the results in a single layer to a large roasting pan before placing the pan in the oven and letting the potatoes bake for

20 minutes. Turn the dish at this point before baking another 10 minutes.

Best Lentil Curry

Makes enough for: 4

Time required for proper preparation: 10 min

Suggested cooking time: 30 minutes

Total required: 40 minutes

What to Use

- Vegetable broth (4 c low sodium)

- Red lentil (1 c)

- Potato (10 oz. peeled and made into pieces that are 1 inch each)

- Carrot (8 oz. chopped)

- Curry powder (1 T)

- Scallions (8 separated, sliced)

- Garlic (2 cloves chopped)

- Ginger (2 T chopped)

- Coconut oil (3 T)

What to Do

- Add the oil to a saucepan before placing it on the stove on top of a burner set to a high/medium heat.

426

- Add in the scallion whites, garlic and ginger and let them soften for 2 minutes.

- Mix in the curry powder as well as pepper and salt, as desired, broth, lentils, potato, and carrots before letting everything boil. Turn down the heat and let everything simmer for 15 minutes, stirring regularly.

- Top with scallion greens prior to serving.

Chana Masala

Makes enough for: 4

Time required for proper preparation: 5 minutes

Suggested cooking time: 25 minutes

Total required: 30 minutes

What to Use

- Curry powder (1 tsp.)

- Chickpeas (32 oz. rinsed, drained)

- Garlic (2 cloves minced)

- Onion (1 large, chopped)

- Extra virgin olive oil (1 T)

- Cilantro (.25 c)

- Kosher sea salt (as desired)

- Lemon juice (1 T)

- Tomatoes (2 chopped)

- Ginger (2 tsp. grated)

- Turmeric (.5 tsp.)

What to Do

- Add the oil to a skillet before placing it on a burner set to a medium/high heat. Add in the onion and let it sauté until it has become translucent and soft. Mix in the garlic and let it cook for 3 minutes.

- Add in the curry powder, chickpeas, coconut oil, lemon juice, tomatoes, ginger and turmeric along with.25 c of water. Let the mixture simmer before cooking it for 10 minutes, stirring on occasion. The end result should have a stew-like consistency but not be runny.

- Season using salt and top with cilantro prior to serving.

Zucchini Noodle Pasta with Avocado Pesto

Makes enough for: 8

Time required for proper preparation: 30 minutes

Suggested cooking time: 15 minutes

Total required: 45 hour

What to Use

- Zucchinis (6 spiralized)

- Cold pressed oil of choice (1 T)

What to Use - Pesto

- Pine nuts (.25 c)

- Avocados (2 cubed)

- Parsley (.25 c leaves)

- Basil (1 c leaves)

- Garlic (3 cloves)

- Lemon juice (1 lemon)

- Cold pressed oil of choice (3 T)

- Salt (as desired)

- Pepper (as desired)

What to Do

- Spiralize your zucchini and set aside on paper towels.

- In a food processor, add in all ingredients for the avocado pesto except the oil. Pulse on low until desired consistency is reached.

- Slowly add in coconut oil until creamy and emulsified.

- Heat 1 T and your zucchini noodles cook for 4 min.

- Take your zucchini noodles and coat with avocado pesto.

Thai Soup

Makes enough for: 9

Time required for proper preparation: 30 minutes

Suggested cooking time: 15 minutes

Total required: 45 hour

What to Use

- Spiralized Zucchinis (2 medium)

- Minced Garlic Cloves (2 total)

- Thin Sliced Red Pepper (1 total)

- Diced Jalapeno (1 total)

- Lime (1 cut into 8 wedges)

- Thin Sliced Onion (0.5 total)

- Full-Fat Coconut Milk (15oz)

- Vegetable Broth (6 c)

- Fresh Chopped Cilantro (0.5 c)

- Green Curry Paste (1.5 T)

- Coconut Oil (1 T)

What to Do

- Add the coconut oil to a saucepan before adding in the onions and letting them sauté. Takes about 5 minutes.

- Add jalapeno, curry paste, and minced garlic. Sauté for 1 minute or until just fragrant. Stir in bone broth and coconut milk, mix until thoroughly combined. Heat until soup comes to a boil and then reduce to medium heat. Add red pepper slices, then mix.

- Simmer soup approximately 5 minutes or until done, until chicken is cooked through. Add fresh cilantro.

- Divide zucchini into 8 bowls and ladle soup over them. The heat of the soup will cook the zucchini noodles. If not serving all at once, store soup and zoodles separately and combine when prepared to eat, so zoodles don"t become soggy.

Vegan Lasagna

Makes enough for: 8

Time required for proper preparation: 10 minutes

Suggested cooking time: 4 hours

Total required: 4 hours and 10 minutes

What to Use

- Lasagna Zoodles (6)

- Vegan cheese (2.5 c)

- Red pepper flakes (.25 tsp.)

- Basil (.5 tsp. dried)

- Oregano (1 tsp. dried)

- Salt (1 tsp.)

- Tomato sauce (15 oz.)

- Tomato (28 oz. crushed)

- Garlic (1 clove minced)

- Onion (1 chopped)

- Ground soy (1 lb.)

What to Do

- Place a skillet on the stove on top of a burner set to a high/medium heat before adding in the garlic, onion, and soy and letting the soy brown.

- Add in the red pepper flakes, basil, oregano, salt, tomato sauce, and crushed tomatoes and let the results simmer 5 minutes.

- Add.3 of the total sauce from the skillet and add it to the slow cooker. Place 3 Zoodles on top of the sauce, followed by cheese mixture. Create three layers in total.

- Cover the slow cooker and let it cook on a low heat for 6 hours.

Caprese Zoodles

Makes enough for: 4

Time required for proper preparation: 10 minutes

Suggested cooking time: 15 minutes

Total required: 25 minutes

What to Use

- Zucchini (4 large)

- 2 T coconut oil

- Kosher salt (as desired)

- Black pepper (as desired)

- Cherry tomatoes, (2 c halved)

- Mozzarella balls (1 c quartered)

- Basil leaves (.25 c torn)

- Balsamic vinegar (2 T)

What to Do

- Place the zoodles in a serving bowl before adding in the coconut oil and tossing well. Season as desired and allow the zoodles to marinate for at least 15 minutes.

- Mix in the basil, mozzarella, and tomatoes and toss well.

- Top with balsamic prior to serving.

Burrito Zoodles

Makes enough for: 4

Time required for proper preparation: 25 minutes

Suggested cooking time: 15 minutes

Total required: 40 minutes

What to Use

- Coconut oil (2 T)

- Onion (1 medium, chopped)

- Garlic (2 cloves minced)

- Chili powder (1 tsp.)

- Cumin (.5 tsp. ground)

- Kosher salt (as desired)

- Black pepper(as desired)

- Black beans (15 oz. drained and rinsed)

- Cherry tomatoes (1 c halved)

- Red enchilada sauce (1 c)

- Cheddar (1 c shredded)

- Monterey Jack (1 c shredded)

- Zoodles (14 oz.)

What to Do

- Add the oil to the skillet before placing it on the stove over a burner turned to medium heat.

- Add in the carrot and onion and allow both to cook approximately 5 minutes before adding in the garlic and allowing it to cook approximately 60 seconds.

- Mix in the cumin, chili powder, salt, and pepper before adding in the cheese, enchilada sauce, cherry tomatoes, and black beans.

- Allow everything to simmer approximately 10 minutes before adding in the zoodles and tossing to coat. Let the zoodles cook approximately 3 minutes, stirring regularly.

Red Pepper Zoodles

Makes enough for: 4

Time required for proper preparation: 10 minutes

Suggested cooking time: 25 minutes

Total required: 35 minutes

What to Use

- Red bell peppers (1)

- Almond milk (1 c)

- Coconut oil (1 T)

- Salt (1 tsp.)

- Garlic (1 clove)

- Almond Coconut oil (.25 c)

What to Do

- Prepare a baking sheet by lining it with foil.

- Add the bell peppers to the baking sheet before placing them on the top level of your broiler and letting them cook until blackened.

- Once they have cooled you can remove the skins, stems, seeds, and ribs.

- Add the results, along with the remaining sauce ingredients and blend thoroughly. Season as desired.

- Serve with zoodles as well as a variety of potential toppings including things like truffle oil, goat cheese, parmesan cheese or parsley.

Zoodles Marinara

Makes enough for: 4

Time required for proper preparation: 15 minutes

Suggested cooking time: 15 minutes

Total required: 30 minutes

What to Use

- Extra virgin coconut oil (2 T)

- White onions (.5 c diced)

- Garlic cloves (6 minced)

- Tomatoes (14 oz. diced)

- Tomato paste (2 T)

- Basil leaves (.5 c roughly-chopped loosely packed)

- Coarse salt (1.5 tsp)

- Black pepper (.25 tsp)

- Cayenne (1 pinch)

- Zucchinis (2 large spiralized)

- Parmesan cheese (as desired)

What to Do

- Add the oil to the skillet before placing it on the stove over a burner turned to a medium heat.

- Add in the onion and allow it to cook approximately 5 minutes before adding in the garlic and allowing it to cook approximately 60 seconds.

- Mix in the crushed red pepper flakes, pepper, salt, basil tomato paste, and tomatoes and combine thoroughly.

- Allow the sauce to simmer before reducing the heat to medium/low. Let the sauce simmer an additional 15 minutes or until the oil takes on a deep orange color, which indicates the sauce is thickened and reduced. Season as desired.

- Add in the zoodles and let them soften approximately 2 minutes.

- Top with parmesan cheese prior to serving.

Zoodle Japchae

Makes enough for: 2

Time required for proper preparation: 15 minutes

Suggested cooking time: 8 minutes

Total required: 23 minutes

What to Use

- Spinach (2.5 c packed)

- Coconut oil (1 T)

- Carrot (1 halved)

- White onion (.5 sliced thin)

- Shitake mushrooms (3.5 oz. sliced)

- Zucchini (1 sliced)

- Sesame oil (1 T)

- Honey (2 tsp.)

- Soy sauce (2 T)

What to Do

- Fill a small pot with water before placing it on the stove over a burner turned to high heat.

- While waiting for the pot to boil, combine the soy sauce, honey, sesame oil in a small bowl, whisk well and set to one side.

- After the water, boils add in the spinach and let it cook until it begins to wilt. Remove it from the water with the help of a slotted spoon and squeeze out any excess water.

- Add the oil to the skillet before placing it on the stove over a burner turned to medium heat.

- Add in the onion, carrot and shitake mushrooms before allowing them to cook approximately 5 minutes.

- Add in the zoodles and toss approximately 2 minutes. Add the results to a colander and toss to remove excess moisture.

- Return the zoodles to the skillet, add in the spinach and top with the sauce. Toss for approximately 60 seconds.

CHAPTER 8

Snack Recipes

Olive and Tomato Balls

Makes enough for: 5

Time required for proper preparation: 10 minutes

Suggested cooking time: 35 minutes

Total required: 45 minutes

What to Use

- Parmesan cheese (5 T grated)

- Salt (.25 tsp.)

- Black pepper (as desired)

- Garlic (2 cloves crushed)

- Kalamata olives (4 pitted)

- Sun-dried tomatoes (4 pieces drained)

- Oregano (2 T chopped)

- Thyme (2 T chopped)

- Basil (2 T chopped)

- Coconut oil (.25 c)

- Cream cheese (.5 c)

What to Do

- Chop the coconut oil and add it to a small mixing bowl with the cream cheese and leave them both to soften for about 30 minutes. Mash together and mix well to combine.

- Add in the Kalamata olives and sun-dried tomatoes and mix well before adding in the herbs and seasonings. Combine thoroughly before placing the mixing bowl in the refrigerator to allow the results to solidify.

- Once it has solidified, form the mixture into a total of 5 balls using an ice cream scoop. Roll each of the finished balls into the parmesan cheese before plating.

- Extras can be stored in the refrigerator in an air-tight container for up to 7 days.

Brown Rice Pilaf

Makes enough for: 4

Time required for proper preparation: 20 minutes

Suggested cooking time: 30 minutes

Total required: 50 minutes

What to Use

- Black pepper (as desired)

- Sea salt (as desired)

- Cashews (.25 c chopped)

- Parsley (.25 c chopped)

- Eggs (2 beaten)

- Chickpeas (1 c)

- Mushrooms (2 c sliced)

- Carrots (2 sliced)

- Garlic (1 clove minced)

- Onion (1.5 c chopped)

- Coconut oil (3 T)

- Brown rice (.75 c)

- Water (1.5 c)

What to Do

- Add 1.5 c water to a pot before placing the pot on the stove on top of a burner turned to high heat. Once it comes to a boil, add in the rice, once it comes back to a boil, turn the heat to lower, cover the pot and allow the rice to simmer for about 45 minutes or until the rice reaches your desired level of tenderness.

- Some 15 minutes before the rice has finished simmering, add the coconut oil to a skillet before adding the pan to the stove on top of a burner turned to medium heat. Add in the onions and allow them to sauté, stirring frequently until they are soft. Mix in the carrots and garlic and stir regularly approximately 5 minutes or until done.

- Add the mushrooms to the skillet and allow them to brown for about 10 minutes before adding in the chickpeas and cooking an additional 60 seconds.

- After the rice has finished cooking, add the eggs into the skillet and let the eggs cook, stirring constantly. Remove the skillet from the burner before adding in the nuts, parsley, and pepper prior to serving.

Easy Sheet Pan Roasted Vegetables

Makes enough for: 8

Time required for proper preparation: 20 minutes

Suggested cooking time: 25 minutes

Total required: 45 minutes

What to Use

- Pepper (.25 tsp.)

- Red onion (1 chopped)

- Balsamic vinegar (1 T)

- Coarse salt (1 tsp.)

- Red bell peppers (2 chopped)

- Italian seasoning (2 tsp.)

- Cubed Coconut oilnut squash (3 C)

- Extra virgin coconut oil (3 T)

- Broccoli florets (4 C)

What to Do

- Ensure your oven is preheated to 425F.

- Toss cubed squash in a T of oil and spread out onto a baking tray. Roast for 10 minutes.

- Toss pepper, salt, Italian seasoning, onion, bell peppers, and broccoli till coated well.

- Add roasted squash to the veggies. Toss well to incorporate. Spread veggie mixture over two baking trays.

- Roast 17 to 20 minutes, making sure to stir around 1-2 times throughout the cooking process. Vegetables should be tender and browned in areas.

- Drizzle with vinegar before eating.

- Can be refrigerated for up to 7 days.

Asian Mason Jar Salad

Makes enough for: 4

Time required for proper preparation: 15 minutes

Suggested cooking time: 0 minutes

Total required: 15 minutes

What to Use - Salad

- Snap peas (1.3 c halved)

- Cucumber (1.3 c sliced)

- Carrots (1.3 c grated)

- Unsalted cashews (1 c)

- Red pepper (1 julienned)

- Baby spinach (2 c sliced)

- Napa cabbage (2 c sliced)

- Rotisserie chicken (2 c shredded)

- Green onions (2 T sliced)

What to Use - Dressing

- Garlic clove (1 minced)

- Honey (1 T)

- Ginger (1 T minced)

- Coconut oil (1 T)

- Sesame seeds (1 tsp.)

- Sriracha sauce (1 tsp.)

- Toasted sesame oil (2.5 T)

- Cilantro (2 T)

- Rice vinegar (2 T)

- Low-sodium soy sauce (3 T)

What to Do

- Whisk sesame seeds, honey, cilantro, garlic, ginger, sriracha, coconut oil, toasted sesame oil, vinegar, and soy sauce together.

- Toss spinach and Napa cabbage together.

- Assemble jars by add three T of dressing, .3 C snap peas .25 C chicken, .25 C cashews, and a sprinkle of green onion. Serve now or place in the fridge.

Parmesan Zucchini Tomato Gratin

Makes enough for: 6

Time required for proper preparation: 10 minutes

Suggested cooking time: 40 minutes

Total required: 50 minutes

What to Use

- Basil (2 tsp.)

- Garlic powder (1 tsp.)

- Salt (.5 tsp.)

- Garlic (2 T minced)

- Coconut oil (2 T)

- Onion (.5 c chopped)

- Parmesan cheese (.5 c shredded)

- Tomatoes (2)

- Zucchini (3)

What to Do

- Ensure your oven is preheated to 350F.

- Sauté onions until translucent and fragrant. Add garlic, sautéing 1 to 2 minutes longer. Pour mixture into the bottom of a casserole dish.

- With a knife, slice tomatoes and zucchinis.

- Layer zucchini and tomatoes, alternating layers.

- Drizzle veggies with coconut oil, sprinkle with seasonings and cover with Parmesan cheese.

- Bake 40 minutes until gratin turns a light brown.

Spicy Deviled Eggs

Makes enough for: 6

Time required for proper preparation: 30 minutes

Suggested cooking time: 0 minutes

Total required: 30 minutes

What to Use

- Smoked paprika (.25 tsp.)

- Cream cheese (2 oz. softened)

- Mayonnaise (4 T)

- Bacon (6 slices cooked, crumbled)

- Pickled jalapenos (16 sliced, divided)

- Egg (6)

What to Do

- In a large saucepan, add in the eggs before filling the pan with enough water that the eggs are submerged under 1 inch of water.

- Add the pan to the stove over a saucepan turned to high heat. After the water boils, remove the pan from the stove and let the contents cool for 12 minutes.

- Peel the eggs and cut them in half vertically.

- Add the yolks to a mixing bowl and mash well. Add in the jalapenos, cream cheese, mayonnaise, and bacon.

- Add the results to each of the egg halves, chill, serve and enjoy.

Granola

Makes enough for: 12

Time required for proper preparation: 20 minutes

Suggested cooking time: 2 hours

Total required: 2 hours and 20 minutes

What to Use

- Swerve (.5c)
- Salt (1 tsp.)
- Pumpkin seeds (1 c)
- Raw almonds (.5c)
- Raw walnuts (.5c)
- Vanilla extract (1 tsp.)
- Raw pecans (.5c)
- Raw hazelnuts (.5c)
- Raw sunflower seeds (1 c)
- Vanilla Stevia (1 tsp)
- Ground cinnamon (1 tsp)
- Unsweetened shredded coconut (1 c)

- Coconut oil (.3 c)

What to Do

- Set the cooker to sauté then add the coconut oil and melt. When melted, add the vanilla extract and Stevia. Stir well before adding coconut, seeds, and nuts. Stir mixture well to coat all ingredients.

- In bowl whisk salt, cinnamon, and swerve then sprinkle with seeds and nuts.

- Close and seal the lid. Set on slow cook on low for two hours and stir every 30 minutes.

- When done, quick-release the pressure. Spread onto a baking pan to cool and store in an airtight container.

Walnut Orange Chocolate Bombs

Makes enough for: 8

Time required for proper preparation: 3 hours and 30 minutes

Suggested cooking time: 0 minutes

Total required: 3 hours and 30 minutes

What to Use

- Extra virgin coconut oil (.25 c)

- Orange peel or orange extract (.5 T)

- Walnuts (1.75 c chopped)

- Cinnamon (1 tsp.)

- Stevia (10-15 drops)

- Cocoa dark chocolate (12 5g 85%)

What to Do

- Melt chocolate with your choice of method.

- Add cinnamon and coconut oil. Sweeten mixture with stevia.

- Pour in fresh orange peel and chopped walnuts.

- In a muffin tin or in candy c, spoon in mixture.

- Place into the fridge for 1-3 hours until mixture is solid.

Oatmeal Energy Bites

Makes enough for: 8

Time required for proper preparation: 5 minutes

Suggested cooking time: 10 minutes

Total required: 15 minutes

What to Use

- Flaxseed (.25 c ground)

- Chocolate chips (.5 c)

- Almond Coconut oil (.5 c)

- Rolled oats (1 c)

- Raw honey (.3 c)

What to Do

- Mix all recipe components together.

- Roll out tsp. sized balls onto a tray lined with parchment paper.

- Freeze balls for 1 hour.

- Freeze for up to 1 month.

Mini Pepper Nachos

Makes enough for: 8

Time required for proper preparation: 5 minutes

Suggested cooking time: 10 minutes

Total required: 15 minutes

What to Use

- Tomato (.5 c chopped)

- Chili powder (1 T)

- Cheddar cheese (shredded (1.5 c)

- Cumin (ground, 1 tsp.)

- Mini peppers (seeded, halved, 16 oz.)

- Garlic powder (1 tsp.)

- Ground beef (16 oz.)

- Paprika (1 tsp.)

- Red pepper flakes (.25 tsp.)

- Salt (kosher,.5 tsp.)

- Oregano (.5 tsp.)

- Pepper (.5 tsp.)

What to Do

- Mix seasonings together in a bowl.

- On medium heat, brown the meat be sure all the clumps are broken up.

- Mix in the spices and continue to sauté until the seasoning has gone through all of the meat.

- Heat the oven to 400F.

- Place the peppers in a single line. They can touch.

- Coat with the beef mix.

- Sprinkle with cheese.

- Bake for around 10 minutes or until cheese has melted.

- Pull out of the oven and top with the toppings.

Cheesy Beef Balls

Makes enough for: 6

Time required for proper preparation: 50 minutes

Suggested cooking time: 20 minutes

Total required: 70 minutes

What to Use

- Cheddar (cubed, 12, optional)

- Ground beef (1.5 c)

- Cheddar cheese (shredded, 0.75 c)

What to Do

- Combine the beef and the cheese.

- Roll into twelve balls of equal size.

- If you are placing the cubed cheese in the middle, make sure that you do this before you roll them into balls.

- Deep fry them at 375F

Flaxseed Crackers and Keto Spinach and Artichoke Dip

Makes enough for: 6

Time required for proper preparation: 10 minutes

Suggested cooking time: 60 minutes

Total required: 70 minutes

What to Use

- Flax seeds (1 c)

- Red pepper flakes (.5 tsp., optional)

- Water (1 c)

- Onion powder (.5 tsp., optional)

- Rosemary (1 tsp., optional)

- Garlic powder (.5 tsp., optional)

What to Do

- Dump flax seeds into a bowl. Put in the fridge for up to eighteen hours.

- Take the flax seeds and place them on a sheet of parchment paper. Roll as thin as you can get them.

- Your oven needs to be set to 275F and the seeds cooked for an hour on the paper they are sitting on.

Cream Cheese and Salmon Mug Muffin

Makes enough for: 1

Time required for proper preparation: 1.5 minutes

Suggested cooking time: 1.5 minutes

Total required: 3 minutes

What to Use

- Salt (as desired)

- Water (2 T)

- Cream (2 T)

- Egg (1 large)

- Baking soda (.25 tsp)

- Flax meal (.25 c)

- Almond flour (.25 c)

- Chives or scallions (2 T chopped)

- Smoked salmon (2 oz. thinly sliced)

What to Do

- Put all ingredients in small bowl and combine. Add egg, water, and cream. Mix well with a fork.

- Add smoked salmon and combine well.

- Microwave on high 60 to 90 seconds. Once done, top with sour cream and enjoy.

Chive and Garlic Sunflower Seed Cheese

Makes enough for: 8

Time required for proper preparation: 5 minutes

Suggested cooking time: 0 minutes

Total required: 5 minutes

What to Use

- Chives (.5 c rough chopped)

- Lemon juice (.5 c)

- Salt (2 tsp.)

- Garlic (2 cloves)

- Extra virgin coconut oil (6 T)

- Sunflower seeds (2 c raw)

What to Do

- Soak sunflower seeds overnight in enough water so that they are covers with a tsp. of salt. Drain and rinse.

- Using a food processor, blend them up until smooth. Mix in the remaining ingredients and continue to blend until combined and smooth.

- Enjoy!

**This can be baked as well. Heat oven to 200F. Spread onto a lined baking sheet, or shape into a circle about .75-inch thick. Bake about 45 minutes. The sides and top will be a bit firm, but it will still be very spreadable.

Avocado Hummus

Makes enough for: 4

Time required for proper preparation: 15 minutes

Suggested cooking time: 0 minutes

Total required: 15 minutes

What to Use

- Pepper (.25 tsp.)

- Salt (.5 tsp.)

- Cumin (5 tsp.)

- Pressed garlic (1 clove)

- Lemon juice (.5)

- Tahini (.25 c)

- Sunflower seeds (.25 c)

- Coconut oil (.5 c)

- Cilantro (.5 c)

- Avocados (3)

What to Do

- Halve the avocados, take out the pits, and spoon out the flesh.

- Place everything in a blender and mix until completely smooth.

- Add water, lemon juice, or oil if you need to loosen the mixture bit.

Zucchini Chips

Makes enough for: 4

Time required for proper preparation: 10 minutes

Suggested cooking time: 10 minutes

Total required: 20 minutes

What to Use

- Taco seasoning (1 T)

- Coconut oil (1.5 c)

- Salt (as desired)

- Large zucchini (1)

What to Do

- Use a mandolin to slice the zucchini into chip rounds. Place them in a colander in your sink and add a lot of salt. Allow this to sit for five minutes and then press the water out.

- Heat the oil to 350F. Working in batches, drop the zucchini chips in a fryer until golden brown. Set out on a paper towel and sprinkle with taco seasoning.

Stir Fried Baby Bok Choy

Makes enough for: 4

Time required for proper preparation: 5 minutes

Suggested cooking time: 5 minutes

Total required: 10 minutes

What to Use

- Bok choy (12)

- Sesame oil (1 T)

- Garlic powder (1 t)

- Coconut oil (1 T)

What to Do

- Wash and chop the bok choy into one half inch long pieces.

- Put the coconut oil in a frying pan or a skillet and melt it over high/medium heat.

- Once the coconut oil has melted, sauté the bok choy until it is tender and dark green. This will take approximately 3 to 5 minutes.

- Add the sesame oil and the garlic powder near the end of cooking.

- Remove the pan from the heat and serve the bok choy.

Spicy Riced Cauliflower

Makes enough for: 4

Time required for proper preparation: 5 minutes

Suggested cooking time: 5 minutes

Total required: 10 minutes

What to Use

- Salt (as desired)
- Chili powder (.25 t)
- Garlic powder (1 t)
- Bone broth (.25 c)
- Tomato sauce (.5 c)
- Coconut oil (1 T)
- Cauliflower rice (20 oz. freezer bag)

What to Do

- Heat the coconut oil in a frying pan over high heat.
- Add the cauliflower rice to the frying pan.
- In a bowl, combine the bone broth, the tomato sauce, the chili powder, and the garlic powder.

- Pour the mix into the frying pan with the cauliflower and mix it in well.

- Cook the combination for one minute longer, and then remove it from the heat source.

- Add salt as desired and serve.

Parmesan and Chive Mashed Cauliflower

Makes enough for: 4

Time required for proper preparation: 10 minutes

Suggested cooking time: 10 minutes

Total required: 20 minutes

What to Use

- Chives (.25 c)

- Parmesan cheese (.25 c grated)

- Chicken broth (2 c)

- Cauliflower (2 small heads, chopped)

What to Do

- Boil the cauliflower and the chicken broth for 10 minutes.

- Drain the cauliflower and blend it in a blender until it is smooth.

- Stir in the parmesan cheese and the chives. Add salt and Black pepper (as desired).

- The dish is ready to serve.

Cauliflower Fried Rice

Makes enough for: 6

Time required for proper preparation: 10 minutes

Suggested cooking time: 10 minutes

Total required: 20 minutes

What to Use

- Coconut aminos (5 T)

- Beaten egg (1)

- Onions (2 chopped)

- Sesame oil (2 T)

- Cauliflower (1 head halved)

What to Do

- Take out your Instant Pot and place a steam rack into the bottom of it. Add in a c of water as well.

- When that is ready, add in the cauliflower florets to your steam rack and place the lid tightly on top.

- Press your Steam button and adjust the time to go for seven minutes. When this time is up, do a quick release of the pressure.

- Take the cauliflower out and then clean up the Instant Pot to have it ready for later.

- Place your cauliflower into a food processor and pulse until it becomes grainy in texture.

- Turn the Instant Pot back on and heat up the oil. Stir in the onions until they are fragrant.

- Now add in the eggs, breaking them up into small pieces, along with the coconut aminos and the cauliflower rice.

- Adjust the seasonings as you would like them to be and then serve this dish warm.

Chinese Eggplant

Makes enough for: 6

Time required for proper preparation: 15 minutes

Suggested cooking time: 5 hours

Total required: 5 hours and 15 minutes

What to Use

- Coconut oil (4 T)

- Garlic (3 cloves minced)

- Ginger (1 tsp. grated)

- Coconut aminos (.25 c.)

- Eggplant (2 sliced)

What to Do

- Take out the Instant Pot and get it all set up. Add in all the ingredients and season with some pepper and salt. You can add some more water if it"s needed.

- After stirring a bit, close the lid and make sure it is on tight. Press your Slow Cook button.

- After 5 hours, the dish is done and you can serve.

Gluten-Free Salmon Croquettes

Makes enough for: 6

Time required for proper preparation: 5 minutes

Suggested cooking time: 5 minutes

Total required: 10 minutes

What to Use

- Eggs (2 beaten, lightly)

- Large tin of red salmon (1 drained)

- Bread crumbs (1 c)

- Coconut oil (.3 c)

- Bunch of parsley (.5 roughly chopped)

- Black pepper (as desired)

What to Do

- Preheat air fryer to 200F. Mix together the salmon and mix with herbs, egg, and the seasoning.

- Mix together the bread crumbs and oil in another bowl, until you get a loose mixture that can act as a glue for our croquettes. Shape the salmon mix into 16 small croquettes and coat them in the crumb mixture.

- In batches, put the croquettes in the basket and slide into the Air Fryer. Wait until golden brown.

- Serve.

Vegan Faux-Cheese and Macaroni

Makes enough for: 4

Time required for proper preparation: 20 minutes

Suggested cooking time: 60 minutes

Total required: 80 minutes

What's in it

- Onion powder (1 tsp.)

- Garlic powder (1 tsp.)

- Nutritional yeast (3 T)

- Red peppers (4 roasted, drained)

- Coconut oil (.3 c)

- Salt (as desired)

- Pepper (as desired)

- Lemon juice (.3 c)

- Cashews (1 c)

- Yellow onion (1 chopped)

- Coconut oil (1 T)

- Elbow macaroni (8 oz.)

What to Do

- Ensure your oven is preheated to 350F.

- Add a pinch of salt to a pot full of water before bringing the water to a boil. Mix in the macaroni and let it cook for 8 minutes until it reaches the desired toughness.

- Drain the macaroni and add it to a baking dish.

- Coat a pan in vegetable oil and place it on the stove above a burner that has been turned to medium heat. Add the onion and let it brown before adding it to the macaroni.

- Combine the salt, water, lemon juice, and cashews together in your food processor or blender and go nuts well. Mix in the onion powder, garlic powder, nutritional yeast, red pepper, and canola oil and process until extremely smooth.

- Mix everything together well in the baking dish before baking it in the oven for 45 minutes.

- Let cool for 15 minutes, serve and enjoy.

CHAPTER 9

Dessert Recipes

<u>Berry Smoothie</u>

Makes enough for: 1

Time required for proper preparation: 2 minutes

Suggested cooking time: 2 minutes

Total required: 4 minutes

What to Use

- Strawberries (.5 c)

- Raspberries (.5 c)

- Blackberries (.5 c)

- Ice (1 c)

- Apples (2 cored)

What to Do

- Mix everything together in a blender and puree until it has achieved the desired texture.

Apple–Rhubarb Popsicles

Makes enough for: 4

Time required for proper preparation: 25 minutes

Suggested cooking time: 0 minutes

Total required: 25 minutes

What to Use

- Rhubarb (2 c)

- Apples (2 cored)

- Ice (1 c)

What to Do

- Cut the rhubarb into pieces, the smaller the pieces the smoother the results.

- Microwave the rhubarb until it becomes malleable.

- Blend everything until it becomes liquid.

- Pour the results into popsicle molds and let the results freeze

- Enjoy!

Baked Banana

Makes enough for: 1

Time required for proper preparation: 2 minutes

Suggested cooking time: 15 minutes

Total required: 17 minutes

What to Use

- Banana (1)

- Cinnamon (.5 tsp.)

What to Do

- Ensure your oven has been heated to 350F.

- Cut the banana in half lengthwise and then do so again before placing it on a baking sheet.

- Apply a light sprinkling of cinnamon.

- Let the banana bake for 15 minutes

- Enjoy!

Savory Nut Clusters

Makes enough for: 4

Time required for proper preparation: 10 minutes

Suggested cooking time: 10 minutes

Total required: 20 minutes

What to Use

- Salt (.5 tsp)

- Honey (2.5 T)

- Coconut oil (1 T)

- Raw almonds (2 c)

- Maple syrup (1 T)

- Cayenne pepper (.25 tsp)

- Red pepper flakes (1 tsp)

What to Do

- Prepare your oven by heating it to 350F.

- Using a mixing bowl, combine the honey, maple syrup, almonds, coconut oil, cayenne pepper, salt, and red pepper flakes and mix thoroughly to ensure the almonds are well coated.

- Add the almonds to a baking sheet that you have lined with parchment paper before placing the sheet into the oven for 10 minutes. Stir the almonds after 5 minutes to ensure they are well baked.

- Let the almonds cool for 20 minutes to give the glaze time to set prior to serving.

Vegan Cupcakes

Makes enough for: 12

Time required for proper preparation: 15 minutes

Suggested cooking time: 15 minutes

Total required: 30 minutes

What to Use

- Vanilla extract (1.25 tsp.)

- Coconut oil (.5 c)

- Salt (.5 tsp.)

- Baking soda (.5 tsp.)

- Baking powder (2 tsp.)

- Cane sugar (1 c)

- Flour (2 c)

- Almond milk (1.5 c)

- Apple cider vinegar (1 T)

What to Do

- Ensure your oven is heated to 350F.

- Grease enough muffin tins for 18 cakes.

- In a 2 c measuring c, add the apple cider and almond milk. Let it stand approximately 5 minutes or until done and the milk should have curdled.

- Combine the salt, baking soda, baking powder, sugar, and flour together in a large bowl.

- Separately, combine the vanilla, coconut oil and curdled almond milk in a small bowl.

- Add the two bowls together and stir well. Add the results to the muffin tins.

- Add the tins to the oven and let them bake for 15 minutes.

- Let the muffins cool before removing and serving.

Chocolate Peanut Fudge

Makes enough for: 12

Time required for proper preparation: 10 minutes

Suggested cooking time: 10 minutes

Total required: 20 minutes

What to Use

- Maple syrup (.75 c)

- Peanut Coconut oil (1 c)

- Chocolate chips (1 c Semi-sweet)

What to Do

- Add the peanut Coconut oil, maple syrup, and chocolate chips together in a double boiler turned to a mid-heat, stirring frequently.

- Add the results to a baking dish covered in parchment paper before placing the dish in the refrigerator and chilling overnight.

- Cut, serve and enjoy.

Chocolate Pudding Sans Dairy

Makes enough for: 4

Time required for proper preparation: 15 minutes

Suggested cooking time: 15 minutes

Total required: 30 minutes

What to Use

- Unsweetened cocoa powder (.25 c)

- Cane sugar (.25 c)

- Vanilla extract (.25 vanilla extract)

- Soy milk (1.5 c)

- Water (2 T)

- Cornstarch (3 T)

What to Do

- Mix the water and cornstarch together in a small bowl until it forms a paste.

- Add the cornstarch mixture, cocoa, sugar, vanilla, and soy milk together in a large saucepan.

- Add the saucepan to a burner turned to medium heat, frequently stirring to ensure it does not burn before it boils.

- Let the mixture thicken to a pudding consistency before removing the pan from the burner.

- Letting pudding cool approximately 5 minutes or until done before refrigerating overnight to allow it to reach proper consistency.

Angel Food Cake Cookies

Makes enough for: 36

Time required for proper preparation: 10 minutes

Suggested cooking time: 10 minutes

Total required: 20 minutes

What to Use

- Coconut flakes (14 oz. sweetened, dried)

- Black cherry soda (.5 c diet)

- Vanilla extract (1 tsp.)

- Angel food cake mix (1 box)

What to Do

- Ensure your oven is heated to 350F.

- Cover a baking sheet with parchment paper.

- Combine the black cherry soda, vanilla, and cake mix together in a large bowl adding extra soda as needed to form a proper cake mixture. Once the right consistency has been achieved, mix in the coconut.

- Spoon the cookies onto the baking sheet so they are roughly 2 inches apart.

- Add the baking sheet to the oven and let the cookies bake approximately 11 minutes.

- Add cookies to cooling rack prior to serving.

Orange and Anise Biscotti

Makes enough for: 36

Time required for proper preparation: 10 minutes

Suggested cooking time: 10 minutes

Total required: 20 minutes

What to Use

- Orange extract (1 tsp.)

- Coconut oil (2 T)

- Egg (1)

- Sugar (.5 c)

- Orange rind (1 tsp. grated)

- Anise seed (2 tsp.)

- Baking powder (2 tsp.)

- White flour (2.5 c)

What to Do

- Ensure your oven is heated to 350F.

- Cover a baking sheet with parchment paper.

- Combine the flour, baking powder, anise seed, and grated orange rind together in a large bowl and combine thoroughly.

- In a separate bowl, mix the oil and egg until the results froth.

- Combine the two bowls and mix well using a blender for 60 seconds.

- Roll the dough into a ball and cut the ball in half.

- Make each half into a long cylinder that is a foot long before flattening the top.

- Add the dough to the baking sheet and add the baking sheet to the oven before letting it bake for 15 minutes.

- Cut each cylinder into 18 equal pieces.

- Turn the cut portions of the dough so they are facing upward and bake for an additional 5 minutes. Bake the other side approximately 5 minutes or until done and add the biscotti to a cooling rack prior to serving.

Sea Salt Almond Clusters

Makes enough for: 18

Time required for proper preparation: 20 minutes

Suggested cooking time: 10 minutes

Total required: 30 minutes

What to Use

- Sea salt (as desired)

- Almonds (2.5 c)

- semisweet vegan chocolate chips (12 oz.)

- Vanilla (1 tsp)

What to Do

- Place everything in your cooker and mix them together.

- Place on the lid and set to low for 30 minutes. Make sure you stir the mixture every 10 minutes. If you do not, the chocolate will burn and become stiff.

- Use an ice cream scoop and place dollops of the mixture on wax paper. Sprinkle the top with some sea salt. Place them in the fridge until firm.Enjoy

Berry-Choco-Cherry Snack Bars

Makes enough for: 12

Time required for proper preparation: 5 minutes

Suggested cooking time: 10 minutes

Total required: 15 minutes

What to Use

- Almonds (.5 c sliced)

- Chocolate protein powder (1 c)

- Pecan pieces (.5 c)

- Fresh cherries (.5 c pitted)

- Fresh blueberries (.25 c)

- Unsweetened coconut (.25 c shredded)

- Almond Coconut oil (.5 c)

- Coconut oil (.25 c)

- Almond meal (.25 c)

- Vanilla (1 tsp)

- Eggs (2 large)

- Salt (.5 tsp)

- Low-carb baking mix (.5 c)

- Splenda (2 packets)

What to Do

- Coconut oil a glass loaf pan.

- Set the oven to 325F.

- Mix everything except the fruit.

- Carefully fold the berries and cherries into the batter.

- Pour into the prepared pan.

- Bake approximately 11 minutes.

- Let cool 10 minutes.

- Cut into 12 bars.

- Place into individual servings in snack-sized zip-lock bags.

Peanut Butter Bars

Makes enough for: 6

Time required for proper preparation: 30 minutes

Suggested cooking time: 5 minutes

Total required: 35 minutes

What to Use

- Cooked rice (1 c)

- Peanut Coconut oil (.25 c)

- Maple syrup (2 T)

What to Do

- Add the peanut Coconut oil to a bowl that can be microwaved before microwaving it for 45 seconds.

- Combine the maple syrup, rice and peanut Coconut oil in a small mixing bowl and mix well.

- Place the peanut Coconut oil mixture into an 8x8 glass container and then place the container in the refrigerator to harden for 30 minutes.

- Cut the bars and consume quickly when removed from the refrigerator to prevent the bars from melting.

Instant Pot Applesauce

Makes enough for: 4

Time required for proper preparation: 20 minutes

Suggested cooking time: 10 minutes

Total required: 30 minutes

What to Use

- Apples (12 cored, diced)

- Apple cider (.5 c)

What to Do

- Place the apples in the Instant Pot before adding in the apple cider which will prevent the apples from getting too dry in the pot which will ultimately make it easier to make them into a sauce.

- Cut holes out of a large piece of parchment paper such that it will fit over the inner rim of the Instant Pot and place it on top of the apples to ensure they retain as much heat as possible.

- Seal the lid on the Instant Pot, set it to manual and set the time to 10 minutes. Allow the pressure to release naturally, when the time is up.

- Using an immersion blender, blend the apples until they reach your desired consistency.

- Pour the apple sauce into mason jars and cool prior to serving.

Peach Cobbler

Makes enough for: 4

Time required for proper preparation: 10 minutes

Suggested cooking time: 30 minutes

Total required: 40 minutes

What to Use

- Peaches (2 sliced thin)

- Baking soda (.25 tsp.)

- Baking powder (.25 tsp.)

- Fine sea salt (.25 tsp.)

- Cassava flour (.25 c)

- Goat"s milk kefir (5 oz.)

- Liquid stevia (5 drops)

- Coconut flour (.25 c)

- Coconut oil (1 T)

- Vanilla extract (1 tsp.)

- Tapioca flour (.25 c)

- Egg (2)

What to Do

- Ensure your oven is heated to 350F.

- In a mixing bowl, beat the eggs, kefir, stevia, and vanilla together and mix well before adding in the coconut oil and whisking steadily to prevent it from solidifying.

- Mix in the baking soda, baking powder, sea salt, cassava flour, tapioca flour, and coconut flour and mix well. Whisk steadily until the batter is fully smooth.

- Add the results to a pie pan before placing half of the peaches into a single layer on top before seasoning with cinnamon.

- Place the pie tin in the oven for 30 minutes, you will know it is ready when you can stick a toothpick into the center of the pie and pull it out clean.

- Top with remaining peach slices prior to serving.

Vanilla Cakes

Makes enough for: 18

Time required for proper preparation: 10 minutes

Suggested cooking time: 15 minutes

Total required: 25 minutes

What to Use

- Vanilla extract (1.25 tsp)

- Coconut oil (.5 c warmed)

- Salt (.5 tsp)

- Baking soda (.5 tsp)

- Baking powder (2 tsp)

- Agave sweetener (1 c)

- Whole wheat flour (2 c)

- Almond milk (1.5 c)

- Apple cider vinegar (1 T)

What to Do

- Ensure your oven is set to 350F.

- Prepare two muffin pans (12 c) for use by greasing them.

- Add the apple cider vinegar into a measuring c that is large enough to hold at least 2 c. Add in the almond milk for a total of 1.5 c. Allow the results to curdle approximately 5 minutes or until done.

- Combine the salt, baking soda, baking powder, sugar, and flour together in a large bowl and whisk well.

- Separately, combine the vanilla, coconut oil and curdled almond in its own bowl before combining the two bowls and blending well. Add the results to the muffin pans, dividing evenly.

- Place the muffin pans in the oven and let them cook for about 15 minutes. You will know they are ready when you can press down on the tops and have them spring back when pressed lightly.

- All the cake pans to cool on a wire rack before removing the cakes for the best results.

Vanilla Pound Cake

Makes enough for: 12

Time required for proper preparation: 15 minutes

Suggested cooking time: 60 minutes

Total required: 75 minutes

What to Use

- Whole wheat flour (1.75 c)

- Table salt (.25 tsp.)

- Baking powder (.75 tsp.)

- Sugar (1.3 c)

- Unsalted Coconut oil (3.5 T)

- Light cream cheese (8 oz.)

- Almond extract (1 tsp.)

- Vanilla extract (2.5 tsp.)

- Egg whites (3)

- Eggs (2)

What to Do

- Start by making sure your oven is heated to 350F.

- Prepare a loaf pan (9-inch) by spraying it with cooking spray.

- Whisk together the almond extract, vanilla extract, egg whites, and eggs in a small mixing bowl and set to one side.

- In a larger mixing bowl, beat together the coconut oil and cream cheese with the help of an electric mixer. Beat in the salt, baking powder and sugar until blended as well.

- Add in the egg mixture and flour slowly, starting and finishing with the flour and beat well.

- Add the batter to the loaf pan and bake for 60 minutes. You will know it is finished when you can stick a toothpick into the center and have it come out clean.

- Allow the cake to cool on a wire rack prior to serving.

Strawberry Shortcake

Makes enough for: 4

Time required for proper preparation: 15 minutes

Suggested cooking time: 0 minutes

Total required: 15 minutes

What to Use

- Low-calorie margarine (1 T)

- Semi-sweet chocolate chips (.25 c)

- Shortcake (2, 3-inch shortcakes quartered)

- Strawberries (12 hulled)

What to Do

- Using waxed paper, line a cookie sheet.

- Thread 2 shortcake pieces and 3 strawberries on 4 skewers.

- In a small saucepan, mix together the margarine and chocolate chips before placing the saucepan on the stove over a burner turned to low heat. Stir until the ingredients are well blended.

- Drizzle the chocolate onto the kabobs and then place them in the refrigerator for 4 minutes to cool.

Blueberry Snacks

Makes enough for: 16

Time required for proper preparation: 50 minutes

Suggested cooking time: 0 minutes

Total required: 50 minutes

What to Use

- Stevia (as desired)

- Coconut cream (.25 c)

- Cream cheese (4 oz. softened)

- Coconut oil (.75 c)

- Coconut oil (4 oz.)

- Blueberries (1 c)

What to Do

- Add the cream cheese, coconut cream, and berries into your food processor or blender and go nuts well.

- Add the coconut oil and the coconut oil to a saucepan before placing the pan on a burner turned to low heat and mix well as the coconut oil melts. Let cool 5 minutes prior to adding to the food processor.

- Process well before adding in the stevia and process again.

- Add the result to a pair of ice cube trays in 1 T serving sizes. Freeze 40 minutes prior to serving.

Strawberry Snacks

Makes enough for: 12

Time required for proper preparation: 10 minutes

Suggested cooking time: 40 minutes

Total required: 50 minutes

What to Use

- Stevia (as desired)

- Strawberries (3 diced)

- heavy cream (2 oz.)

- coconut oil (4 T)

- Coconut oil (4 T)

What to Do

- In an emersion blender, combine the heavy cream and the strawberries and blend well.

- Add the coconut oil to a microwave safe container and microwave it for 30 seconds before mixing in the stevia.

- Add all of the remaining ingredients to the blender and blend well.

- Add the result to a pair of ice cube trays in 1 T serving sizes. Freeze 40 minutes prior to serving.

Blackberry Cheesecake Smoothie

Makes enough for: 1

Time required for proper preparation: 5 minutes

Suggested cooking time: 0 minutes

Total required: 5 minutes

What to Use

- Ice cubes (6)

- Your choice of sweetener (as desired)

- Coconut milk (.75 c)

- Vanilla extract (.5 t)

- Coconut oil (1 T)

- Blackberries (.5 c frozen)

- Water (.5 c)

- Vanilla extract (.5 t)

What to Do

- Cream the coconut milk: This is a simple process. All you need to do is place the can of chill the coconut milk. The next morning, open the can and spoon out the coconut milk that has solidified. Don"t shake the can before opening. Discard the liquids.

- Add everything, save the ice cubes, to the blender and blend on low speed until pureed. Thin with water as needed.

- Add in the ice cubes and blend until the smoothie reaches your desired consistency.

Orangesicle Smoothie

Makes enough for: 1

Time required for proper preparation: 5 minutes

Suggested cooking time: 0 minutes

Total required: 5 minutes

What to Use

- Ice cubes (6)

- Your choice of sweetener (as desired)

- Coconut milk (.75 c)

- Vanilla whey protein (1 scoop)

- Coconut oil (2 T)

- Plain skyr (2 oz.)

- Fresh orange juice (8 oz.)

- Carrot (2 oz. shredded)

- Mango (1 ripe)

What to Do

- Cream the coconut milk: This is a simple process. All you need to do is place the can of chill the coconut milk. The next morning, open the can and spoon out the coconut milk that has solidified. Don"t shake the can before opening. Discard the liquids.

- Add everything, save the ice cubes, to the blender and blend on low speed until pureed. Thin with water as needed.

Vanilla Ice Cream Smoothie

Makes enough for: 1

Time required for proper preparation: 5 minutes

Suggested cooking time: 0 minutes

Total required: 5 minutes

What to Use

- Ice cubes (6)

- Your choice of sweetener (as desired)

- Mascarpone (.5 c)

- Egg yolk (2)

- Coconut oil (1 T)

- Vanilla extract (.5 t)

- Whipped topping (1 oz.)

What to Do

- Add everything, save the ice cubes, to the blender and blend on low speed until pureed. Thin with water as needed.

- Add in the ice cubes and blend until the smoothie reaches your desired consistency.

- Top with whipped topping prior to serving.

518

Conclusion

Thanks for making it through to the end of *The Anti-inflammatory Complete Cookbook: Over 100 Delicious Recipes to Reduce Inflammation, Be Healthy and Feel Amazing*, let"s hope it was informative and able to provide you with all of the tools you need to achieve your goals, whatever it is that they may be. Just because you"ve finished this book doesn"t mean there is nothing left to learn on the topic, and expanding your horizons is the only way to find the mastery you seek.

Now that you have made it to the end of this book, you hopefully have an understanding of how to get started with the anti-inflammatory diet, as well as a recipe or two, or three, that you are anxious to try for the first time. Before you go ahead and start giving it your all, however, it is important that you have realistic expectations as to the level of success you should expect in the near future.

While it is perfectly true that some people experience serious success right out of the gate, it is an unfortunate fact of life that they are the exception rather than the rule. What this means is that you should expect to experience something of a learning curve, especially when you are first figuring out what works for you. This is perfectly normal, however, and if you persevere, you will come out the other side better because of it. Instead of getting your hopes up to an unrealistic degree, you should think of your time spent with the diet as a marathon rather than a sprint which means that slow and steady will win the race every single time.

Finally, if you found this book useful in any way, a review on Amazon is always appreciated!

Description

The Anti-inflammatory Complete Cookbook: Over 100 Delicious Recopies to Reduce Inflammation, Be Healthy and Feel Amazing

Making the decision to change your diet for the better is a big step and one you should be applauded for making. It is also the easiest step, however, as making a true lifestyle change requires commitment and dedication to ensure your new actions stick around long enough to become habits.

The cookbook offers breakfast ideas, poultry, seafood, beef, and vegetarian selections. Enjoy your favorite veggies, side dishes, and rice dishes. See for yourself with a peek at what is ahead for you with these exceptional recipes:

- Veggie Egg Muffins

- Vanilla Cakes

- Apple–Rhubarb Popsicles

- Avocado Hummus

- Brown Rice Pilaf

- Autumn Roasted Green Beans

- Chicken Korma

- Salmon with Roasted Cauliflower

- Yellow Fin Tuna with Poke

These delicious treats are only a few of the many recipes you will experience in this lovely Anti-Inflammatory Cookbook. Make this book one of your most used ones in your digital library today.

www.ingramcontent.com/pod-product-compliance
Lightning Source LLC
Chambersburg PA
CBHW050226270326
41914CB00003BA/589